NO MORE
HIDING

NO MORE HIDING

permission to love your sexual self

RHODA LIPSCOMB, PhD.

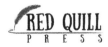

RED QUILL
P R E S S

No More Hiding: Permission to Love Your Sexual Self
Published by Red Quill Press
Castle Rock, CO

Library of Congress Control Number: 2017956260

ISBN: 978-0-9994526-0-8

HEALTH & FITNESS / Sexuality

QUANTITY PURCHASES: Schools, companies, professional groups, clubs, and other organizations may qualify for special terms when ordering quantities of this title. For information, email Rhoda@DrRhoda.com.

♋

This book is dedicated to the many men and women—whether professional client, friend, family member, or even the occasional stranger in the airport—who share with me their fears, challenges, pain, embarrassment, goals and dreams in their quest for answers and direction in their sexual lives. You have all made me a better clinician, author, and advocate for those who want more than the typical sexual and relationship arrangement. My hope is that this book will help guide all of us to better and happier relationships.

Contents

Introduction

Sex and sexuality: even the words cause many people in our Western society to immediately tense up. We have been taught that the mere mention of the subject is taboo and a simple conversation on the subject is in poor taste. Why? Sexuality starts when life starts and runs throughout our lifespan. It is an innate part of the human condition, a part of every human's personality, and what many feel is a sacred part of our birthright.

If society has made it difficult for people to talk in general about sex, imagine how much more difficult it is to talk about sex and sexuality that is considered different or atypical. Those who are considered different may feel even more need to hide who they are, what they want, and the questions that swirl around in their heads. By "different," I don't mean people who want to have sex with the lights on someplace other than the bed after the news is done, or who wish their partner would just know what they desire without having to tell them. The type of different I am talking about is usually not discussed in your typical book on sex. If words like kink, fetish, bondage, or multiple partners pique your interest more than another night of sex in the missionary position, then keep reading; you are on the right track.

This book was created from the exploration and journeys of people who blazed the trails of sexual variety. Their stories are here to show you the way. You will learn what they learned in order to make these unique lifestyles successful. It is designed for those who feel confused, who lack a voice to admit what they desire as well as the strength to explore new sexual trails. It is also designed for those who know what they want, yet lack the tools to get past their fear, shame, and embarrassment. This book has been written for the people who seek more, yet have doubts about leaving the path everyone has told them is the right one. While people have been exploring alternative sexuality for thousands of years, most people in our society have been taught that there is only one right way to engage in intimate relationships, when in reality there are many sexual and relationship styles that people throughout history have used in successful and healthy ways. There are a wide range and variety of sexual activities that people enjoy, from the typical and familiar to unique and atypical behaviors. There can be a great deal of shame and embarrassment about atypical sexual behaviors. However, as long as they are consented to by all involved, they are not bad, wrong, or immoral; they are just different.

As a sexuality professional, I have spent more than 30 years studying the subject, and more than 25 years helping men and women accept sex as a natural part of life. I am also a human being who has spent a lifetime learning to understand and accept my own sexuality.

I know this subject well. This book contains information from my three core areas of knowledge: my academic knowledge - learning from books and teachers; my professional clinical knowledge—the things I have learned from working with thousands of individuals; and my personal knowledge from friends, family members and personal experience. The combination of all three areas makes the journey within the pages of this book more in-depth and well-rounded than any one area could.

We will talk about different relationship styles and how you need to adopt different mindsets in order to successfully navigate these styles, because thinking from traditional relationship mindsets will usually result in failure and frustration. We will also explore various ways of enjoying your sex life, which inevitably relates to shifts in your sexuality as a whole because alternative means of sexual expression also mean your sexuality as a whole shifts (we'll learn more about this in later chapters). We will explore behaviors that are rather sex-specific and other areas that relate more to sexuality.

Sex and sexuality are actually similar, yet different things. Sex relates to the specific sexual acts that human beings and animals engage in, either in pairs, groups or solo. Sexuality is much more difficult to define. Some will define it as an attitude or capacity for sexual feelings. Others confuse sexuality with sexual orientation, which has historically come to mean the genders that one is attracted to—men, women, or both. As someone with a doctoral degree in clinical sexology, my professional experience has led me to define sexuality differently. I tend to see sexuality as an integral and unique part of an individual's personality. It is part of how we react, even how we dress, talk, move and interact with others around us. Sexuality is far more than specific sexual behaviors and often runs deep in our souls. It is light and dark, giving and selfish, and can bring out our best and our worst. It comforts us, excites us, frightens us, brings us together and tears us apart. No wonder we are so confused as a society. We may wonder why others are so afraid of their sexuality; however, when we consider the power it commands, it is not really that surprising.

For those who desire something different or a unique sexuality, allowing oneself to explore this new world can evoke many negative emotions. There is the fear of rejection, a feeling of shame that one is wrong for even having such desires, and the fear of losing a current relationship or being able to find someone else who shares similar desires. The negative emotions of fear, shame, guilt and embarrassment are often very strong when thinking about making this type of life change. Throughout the book we will be addressing these emotions, encouraging you to dig deeper to better understand them, as well as giving you ways to let go of the stranglehold these emotions may currently have on your desire for more from your sexual life. Understanding and getting better control of these emotions may seem like a daunting task, but it's very possible, and I will show you how.

When you take this journey with me, learning to accept and love your sexual self will be the eventual destination. There are some of you who have the desires, yet after reading this book will decide that going on this journey is too much change for you, or at least that you are not at a place in your life where you are ready to make this type of change. Let me tell you now, that is OK. This type of transformation is not for everyone. Yet for those who seek help and permission to explore unique areas of sexuality and relationship dynamics, this will be a very rewarding journey. The book is designed so that along the way there is education about the emotions you may feel, information about where some of the beliefs you currently have about sex came from, and discussion about the various forces in our society that don't want you to break out of your current way of thinking and behaving. We will also cover more in-depth information about

BDSM (bondage and discipline, dominance and submission and sadomasochism), fetishes, kinks and the wide world of open relationships. There are exercises along the way to help you gain greater insight into your desires and emotions and help keep you on track. The initial chapters are devoted to giving you a better overall understanding of the history and background of a society that is set up and works to keep people from exploring alternative sexual expression. The middle chapters are designed to help you grow. The final chapters are written to help you move forward with the changes you decide to make. When you have finished with this journey you will have gained more confidence in yourself, learned to accept and love your true sexuality, and discovered techniques to help you manage the negative emotions of fear, shame, guilt and embarrassment. You will learn to listen to your own inner voice and become authentic with who you are and what you need to live your sexual life fully. You will also be poised and equipped to continue with more exploration if that is what you want.

I have seen many individuals and couples make the transition from fearful and ashamed of their true sexual selves to confident, happy and fulfilled. While sometimes relationships have to end and new ones must be discovered in order for people to be authentic, I have seen many people who have completely surprised me with their willingness to join their partners on unique sexual journeys rather than lose a relationship that holds great importance for them.

I will not lie to you. This journey is not for the meek or those who lack inner strength. It can be a difficult and challenging path, yet one that can also reap great rewards for those who see it through. Many wonder if they truly have that inner strength to take on such a life change, and while not everyone has it, many have been pleasantly surprised to discover that they have far more strength and courage than they realized they had. My guess is that you also have this strength and courage, otherwise you would not have come this far. Please know that you are not alone on this path. There are many others out in the world who seek similar areas of fulfillment; through this book, I will be with you each step of the way. So if you are tired of waiting, tired of wondering what could be, wondering if you are OK, even though you feel differently, then come with me and I will share this amazing new world with you. The next steps are up to you.

Chapter One

The Fork in the Road
Is this really all there is?

David sat in my office, fidgeting in his seat. This was his first appointment with me and while he had spent most of the session making what is considered appropriate eye contact, his gaze suddenly dropped to the floor as he finally talked about what really brought him in to see me. He nervously admitted that he had started a secret life and didn't know how to tell his wife of 15 years, or what to do about it. He knew his wife suspected that something was going on, so he needed to understand what he was doing before he attempted to explain it to her. David had found an online community where he was able to explore the types of sexual interactions which up until recently, he had only fantasied about. Through this website he was interacting with other people through avatars. This made me the first human he had ever told face-to-face about having these feelings and engaging in these activities. Needless to say, he was terrified, embarrassed and slightly ashamed. He was a highly-educated, very successful corporate executive married to an equally educated and successful woman. Friends thought they had it all. So why was he seeking something else? David wondered if there was something wrong with him.

That is often how it starts. People ask themselves, how did I get here? I did everything "right," the way family, friends, and society told me to do it. I married the nice safe guy or girl, and yet I feel like a part of me is dying inside. What is wrong with me? Can you fix me? Or am I just some sort of freak?

As a therapist who specializes in sexuality with a niche in alternative means of sexual expression, I have heard this more times than I care to count. And because I am known for working within this unique area of human sexuality, I hear it from not only the people I see professionally, but from colleagues, friends and family.

Most people feel that sex and relationships shouldn't be so difficult. They have a nagging feeling that sex should be fun and exciting like it was in the beginning. They are bored with their sex lives, often view porn to get some variety, and might buy a vibrator to really spice things up. They want something more, yet not *that* different from the norm.

Let's be clear: this book is not for those people. There are plenty of other sex books out there for monogamous, vanilla-sex people. While we're at it, let's be clear about something else: "vanilla" is not meant as an insult. Instead, it is a descriptive term often used by those in sexually adventurous communities who consider themselves more "rocky road" or some variation of swirl, than typical vanilla. There is nothing wrong with vanilla, rocky road, or chocolate swirled with raspberry sorbet and sprinkles on top. All are valid and OK, just different.

Despite many advances from the sexual revolution decades ago, most of us are still taught the typical societal beliefs about sex and relationships. Monogamy is usually thought of as the only "real" way adult relationships work. And while sex is important in a relationship, it is also just something people do from time to time, especially after you have children. Most of us are also taught that sex is not supposed to be that important as a relationship goes on. It is better and more mature to focus on other aspects of the relationship and give up the need for passion, variety and adventure. Even in situations where the people in the relationship are completely mismatched sexually, we are taught that love conquers all. And as hard as it is to believe, many people still believe that as we get older, we no longer want or care about sex. It doesn't matter that studies show that many healthy individuals care very much about sex later in life, and that people who *do* have an active sex life as they grow older enjoy life more.

Many would say this sounds a bit old fashioned—a 1950s mentality about sex. Unfortunately, for all of the changes and forward movement we have seen among many populations, there are still people for whom this type of thinking is very much alive. It's also what they teach the next generation. I am often shocked by the questions I get about sex in my professional practice that still mirror many of these thoughts. And this level of sexual ignorance is from well-educated people!

Within the last few decades, most of the children in our public schools received abstinence only-sex education, which was more about keeping them afraid of sex, pregnancy and sexually-transmitted infections than real sexual knowledge. Unless they were lucky enough to have parents who gave them accurate information, they learned fear and ignorance rather than the positive aspects of natural pleasure or exploration. So while there have been many advances in sexual knowledge, that is not what many people are learning at this point in the twenty-first century.

This book is designed for people who wonder about different types of sexual lives, the ones lived by "people they hear about." Are those people truly happy? Can these kinds of things be done successfully? How do I get there? It is designed for the people standing at that fork in the road wondering, "Do I stay on the same path I've been on for years, where at least I know what to expect? Or do I take the risk and explore a daring new path?" There can be great fear connected with exploring a new path, including questions like "Will I really be happier? Am I fooling myself? What will people think? Will I lose everything I have worked so hard to attain?"

Throughout this book I will have many roles: part therapist, helping you better understand and process difficult emotions; part coach, encouraging you to work harder and push yourself further; part tour guide, giving you an insider's look at some of the more common alternative sexuality communities; and part confidant, allowing you to process your private thoughts and feelings. We will explore the areas of BDSM (bondage and discipline, dominance and submission, sadomasochism), fetishes, kink and the wide world of open relationships, including polyamory and swinging. Throughout the process I will share stories of real people who have been through the same situations you may be facing. I have changed their names and actual circumstances to protect their identities, but the core aspects of their stories will teach you and help you know that you are not alone in your thoughts and desires. They have taken that other fork in the road and have lived to tell about it.

You are not alone. Other people in the world are feeling or have felt the same as you do now. By mid-life, many people who have done everything they were told was right have worked with therapists or read multiple self-help books. They have made many failed attempts to lessen the feelings of distance from their spouse, especially when it comes to sex. Many would prefer to look at porn rather than feel obligated to engage in the same old dull, lifeless sex they have been having for years.

Still, they wonder what is wrong with them. After all, others seem to be happy with the status quo. Why aren't they? They must be the one with the problem. They secretly wonder if there is something wrong with them for wanting more sexually. Often they feel afraid, ashamed, and embarrassed to admit what they really desire.

Many people are very clear about what they want and desire. They have secretly been engaging in these behaviors for many years. Other people know that they desire more, yet have only a vague and nagging notion of what they need. They fear exploring the unknown and have no idea how to go about breaking out of their shell to be their authentic sexual selves.

It is easy to stay where you are; you don't have to risk the failure you fear. However, there is a price for staying stuck, just as there is a price for change. Whatever decision you make, remember that knowledge is power.

Let's look at a few people who experienced the same early phase of questioning their sexual desires you are feeling now. We will continue to follow their stories throughout the book and share how they progressed through their journey so you get a full picture of what this can look like from beginning to completion. Some have very successful outcomes; and while others do not have quite the Hollywood or fairytale ending, they do have resolution.

David

We started this chapter talking about his journey. He was eventually able to share his issue with me: he had always had what he considered "dark desires" for dominance and submission. This was long before the 50 Shades book and film series had taken the public by storm with romanticized stories of those dark desires. He had kept his dark desires hidden from his very prim and proper wife and was terrified that if she really knew who he was, what he desired, as well as the things he enjoyed having his avatar engage in with other avatars, she would certainly reject and divorce him. He stated that she had discovered the games he was playing online, late one night and had accused him of cheating. He was unsure if he was really cheating since he had not actually met any of the people who were on the other side of his computer screen. However, he was spending more and more hours, late at night engaging with other avatars rather than with his flesh and blood wife. He admitted that he enjoyed these themes of being sexually dominant with women who chose to submit to him; well, at least their avatars submitted to him. He questioned if he could actually do these things in real life. He was certain his wife would never engage in these activities with him. Even though he had felt this way for over 20 years, he wondered if these desires might eventually go away.

Josh

Like David, Josh came to see me to help him understand a fetish he admitted he had enjoyed most of his life. He was sexually aroused by women's feet and shoes, especially high-heeled shoes. He and his wife had been married 12 years and had two young children who he loved very much. Initially he said that his wife enjoyed the attention he paid to her feet when they were having sex in the early years of their marriage, and he thought they had been doing well in their marriage and sex life. This suddenly changed when she found him looking at a women's shoe catalog and realized that he found other women's feet and shoes attractive, not just hers. She accused him of having a sex addiction and refused to allow him to play with her feet sexually any longer. This was very difficult for Josh, because it was an important and fun part of their sex life. Some people with a fetish need it to be involved in order to become sexually aroused. Josh could still function sexually, yet the fun and thrill that had been there earlier in their sex life was gone and all that he was left with was boring sex; same positions, same time of day, same old, same old. He admitted that he would meet other women when he would go out with friends for a drink at a bar, who let him play with their feet and while he had not "technically cheated" he felt guilty about these interactions. He feared his wife would discover what he occasionally did in order to get his needs met, that she would divorce him and take his kids away from him.

Veronica

Veronica was depressed and torn. She was 44, attractive, had recently finished her master's degree, was working as a therapist, and had been married for five years to her second husband. She was a professional colleague and friend of mine, so she felt comfortable confiding in me. This was the second marriage for both her and her husband Michael, and in all areas but one, it was a great marriage. This was the first relationship she had experienced with a man that lasted longer than two years. She frequently left past relationships after a short time because she was bored. And even if she was mostly satisfied, another man began to look sexually interesting and just different. It was important to her to find a way to make this marriage work. Veronica and her husband loved each other deeply, were very compatible as partners and enjoyed each other's company except when it came to sex.

While their sex life had started off strong, it dropped off quickly once the relationship became serious and they made the decision to marry and make a permanent commitment to each other. She found this both confusing and extremely frustrating. She stated that Michael was very physically affectionate and attentive to her, holding hands often and cuddling in bed every night, yet sex was allusive. After five years of marriage, they were having sex approximately once a year, usually after she pointed out to him how long it had been. Michael appeared to have sex out of obligation more than true desire.

It was not surprising that Veronica was depressed, angry, resentful and very frustrated. She had dragged Michael reluctantly to various therapists, couples weekend workshops, and given him numerous books that went unread. Sex had always been a very important part of her life and in her past relationships. She had never experienced a relationship with a man who wasn't interested in her sexually, yet continued to tell her often how attractive and desirable he found her.

Shortly before she met Michael, Veronica was starting to experiment with some sexual variety in her life, even having her first threesome with two men. When she met her new husband, she felt she had to shut down the new things she was enjoying and tried to forget about that time of exploration. When she was being very honest with herself, she knew a threesome with two men was still her favorite sexual fantasy. But now, she felt it had to remain a fantasy.

Michael had told her that he and his ex-wife had experienced a good sex life for 10 years, so what was she doing wrong? Here she was, a therapist helping other people with their relationships, yet she couldn't fix her own. She was tempted to find a lover on the side, yet was afraid that would get too complicated. Veronica didn't know what to do, but knew she had to do something. She couldn't live this way much longer.

Common threads

David, Josh and Veronica are in different situations, but their stories share common threads. All three experience the same negative emotions. For each of them, there is a great deal of fear of losing their partners or being rejected if their partners see their authentic sexual selves. They feel guilt that what they have is not satisfying enough, that they need more, and about how they get (or want to get) their needs met. There is embarrassment for the realization that they are different from their partners, peers and families. And finally, there is shame, one of the most destructive emotions they feel. They are ashamed for being different sexually, as if that means they are flawed, selfish and wrong. Their reactions to these negative emotions cause them to hide their true selves—or their exploration of alternative sexual activity—from their spouses. However, these very explorations are sometimes the only thing that helps them maintain their lives and remain sane. As I often tell my patients, everyone has a breaking point, and it is different for each individual.

How does this relate to you?

While some things we have discussed so far may sound familiar, you also may be wondering how all this relates to you. Most people who are standing at a fork in the road are feeling a wide range of emotions. These can include excited feelings of wanting more along with shame for wanting more, a strong, seemingly overwhelming need for variety, and fear of what might be lost by taking that first step down a new path. Fear is often what stops people and keeps them on the well-worn, comfortable path where they feel safe, even if they are also bored, inauthentic, and resentful that they cannot find the courage to venture to where they feel they belong.

Acknowledging these feelings is really the first step of your journey. Otherwise, these very strong emotions can keep you trapped for a lifetime. They are important to understand but often difficult to learn to manage. That's why the next chapter is devoted to the Big Four emotions: fear, shame, embarrassment, and guilt. We will explore them in more depth, learn how they play a positive role in your life, and understand when they have gotten out of control. I will give you techniques to manage the Big Four so that you can break their power over you.

I have often found that writing is a very strong therapeutic tool that helps people clear their heads and come to a better understanding of difficult areas in their lives. Taking the private thoughts and feelings that run amuck in your head like a bunch of sugared-up preschoolers and putting them down on paper gives you a chance to sort them out. You can see what makes sense with your adult logic and what is just a monster hiding under your bed. I have designed this journey with a number of exercises that allow you to write down your thoughts and feelings in a safe, private way.

Exercise

Answer the following questions and let's see where you are starting your journey. You need to know where you currently are to know how far you have to go.

1. Do you view porn? This can be in visual form on the internet, DVDs, or in magazines; or written form such as classic erotic novels or romance novels; also known as housewife porn. People tend to enjoy the same type of scenarios regardless of the medium. Begin by noticing what your favorite themes are. What scenes do you imagine yourself in? Write those down.

2. Examine your sexual fantasies. Have you gotten to the point where you need to fantasize often in order to function sexually with your partner? If so, what do these fantasies involve?

Additional partners? Special items involved in your sex play? Do you wish you could dominate your partner (tying them to the bed, for example) or do you want to be dominated (having your partner tie you down, for example)? Write these down.

3. Have you ever shared these thoughts with a former or current partner? Was their reaction positive, neutral, negative, or very negative? How did (or does) their reaction affect your feelings of fear, shame, embarrassment, and guilt?

4. How long have you noticed or been able to admit to yourself that you have sexual desires that you think are different from those around you? How long have you been hiding them? What do you think would happen (whether it's accurate or not) if you let these desires out? Notice catastrophic thinking patterns.

Check in: How are you doing?

At the end of each chapter, I will check in with you to see how you are feeling. Throughout the chapters, we will explore deep emotions by way of educational information and exercises designed to stretch and encourage you to really think about who you are, what you want and where you would prefer to be. Since we have just touched on negative feelings that have been holding you back, we will start with some surface-level exploration of your emotions. Don't worry; we will dive much deeper as we go along.

Journal a bit about how you are feeling so far. Are all the emotions you are feeling negative or are there some additional positive or neutral feelings? Begin to notice them, acknowledge them and write them down.

Chapter Two

Negative Emotions

The big four—learning to manage fear,
shame, embarrassment, and guilt

A s human beings, we are bombarded with emotions throughout
the day, week, month and year. They ebb and flow and are a
natural part of being human. Growing up, we're not always given
helpful information about how to deal with our emotions, let alone
the emotions of others. It is no wonder our feelings can overwhelm
us at times.

Positive and negative emotions serve us in many ways, and we
function best when they work together. Many books and philoso-
phies suggest that searching for happiness is the ideal above all else.
This can give people the mistaken belief that all negative emotions
are bad and must be avoided. It leads some people to think that we
should be happy and joyous all the time. However, negative emotions have their place in our emotional balance. Fear can keep us

alert to real danger, such as a wild animal attacking us in the woods. Guilt and shame can keep us from doing truly bad things to other people, like swindling them out of their life savings.

Research shows that as humans, we struggle with our positive and negative emotions. A fascinating study by Dr. Hi Po Bobo Lau from the University of Hong Kong demonstrated that many people would pay large sums of money to avoid strong negative emotions or experience positive emotions more often. In the study, each person was asked to assign a price between $2 and $200 to various emotions. While the opportunity to feel excitement came in at $62.80 and happiness at $79.06, the possibility of avoiding fear registered $83.27; avoiding embarrassment, $99.81; and avoiding regret tallied $106.26. (Kashdan & Biswas-Diener, 2014)

What makes people willing to spend so much money to avoid undesirable emotions? If you think spending money to avoid pain is extreme, I have even had some clients tell me they wish their bad feelings could be surgically removed! We avoid negative emotions for four basic and very intuitive reasons:
1. They are unpleasant.
2. They represent getting stuck in a rut.
3. They are associated with a loss of personal control.
4. They are perceived, correctly, as having social costs.
   (Kashdan & Biswas-Diener, 2014, p. 61)

The four basic reasons for avoiding negative emotions tell us a lot about our hate-hate affair with them. First, we want to avoid feeling crappy because feeling crappy feels crappy. Quite simply, negative emotions are unpleasant and people often underestimate their ability to tolerate the distress of negative emotions.

The second reason is the belief that these feelings are like quicksand—we will get bogged down in them with no hope of escape.

This especially applies to chronic negative emotions such as depression; the thought is these feelings can become permanent.

The third reason we avoid these emotions is we fear that, like a psychological tsunami, they will crash over us and sweep us away to a random, unwanted destination of thoughts and behavior.

Finally, we fear the social consequences of expressing them. While our negative moods do have power, the fear of their power is often over-exaggerated. (Kashdan & Biswas-Diener, 2014)

So, if we can't buy our way out of negative emotions (and clearly, they cannot be surgically removed), what is the best way to deal with them? The truth is that when we learn to accept and manage, rather than avoid, negative emotions, they are useful in keeping us safe and balanced. When we attempt to avoid painful or troubling feelings, they grow and become overwhelming, keeping us stuck in unproductive, unhappy, unsatisfying situations and relationships. On top of that, many parts of our society use the power of these negative emotions as a means of control, which can keep people locked in the shackles of sexual mediocrity. We will focus on this more later in the book, when we explore our ingrained sexual beliefs and the war on men's sexuality.

In this chapter, we will focus on specific emotions that I like to call the Big Four: fear, shame, embarrassment and guilt. When dealing with sexual issues—especially alternative sexual behavior—these four emotions are often a package deal. This makes it appropriate to give most of our attention to them. You have many other feelings; however, because of their power, the Big Four cause the most trouble for many of the people I have worked with professionally. Since you can't really eliminate them, we will discuss ways to better understand these powerful feelings and learn to manage them. This will help you use their power to improve your life rather than suppress and destroy it. I tend to see the latter when people attempt to avoid their emotions rather than face them.

Fear: The big, scary monster in the dark

Everyone is familiar with fear. At some point, we all have been startled by something that caused us to experience fear. It is considered a protective and innate emotion; for example, it is appropriate to be afraid of a wild animal that may attack you in the woods. A small amount of fear helps keep you aware and safe when you're walking down a dark street or driving in heavy traffic. When you experience fear in the moment, bodily functions like your digestive system and sexual functioning shut down so you can use that energy to meet the threat head-on or run away from it. Let's face it, when dealing with a real fear, sexual desire or digesting your food can wait until later. The famed "fight, flight or freeze" phenomenon was first described in 1932 by Harvard physiologist Walter Cannon. It is the most primal of survival mechanisms not only in humans, but virtually all species that have ever been studied for a fear response. (Britten, 2001, p. 20) In these types of situations, fear has a very well-defined and helpful purpose, so eliminating all fear from our lives would be a poor choice indeed.

However, fear that keeps us from attempting things like new sexual behavior becomes more problematic than helpful. All the individuals we discussed in Chapter 1 were experiencing fear of change, fear of rejection, and fear of the unknown. Many of their problems related to fears that required action: deciding to change, asserting themselves, ending a relationship, making a mistake, or becoming truly emotionally intimate with their partners. They also encountered more ego-based fears: rejection, vulnerability, others' disapproval, and being seen as different. And finally, there is what most fear boils down to—people are afraid they can't handle whatever happens. (Jeffers, 2007) I have felt this myself when taking on a new task such as writing this book, and have seen it daily with people I work with professionally. When people come to me to talk about their unique sexual desires, there is usually an enormous amount of fear.

Let me give you an example. One of my long-term clients initially came to me with a unique sexual fetish—wearing a diaper. While his wife was aware of his fetish, she was becoming less and less supportive. During his first visit, my client feared that if he embraced his fetish, his wife would leave him, he would lose his children, his parents and everyone in their conservative small town would discover his secret, and he would be ostracized. As we worked together and he began to accept himself, his wife did file for divorce, sue for full custody of their children, and tell anyone who would listen about his love of wearing diapers (along with other slanderous things that were far from true).

While it would have been easy for him to give into his fears, give her the children, move away, and hide, he didn't. With a lot of support, he faced his fears and got half-time custody of his children. My client was able to continue running a business in his community. He also discovered that his family and true friends were far more supportive and understanding than he could have imagined. This was only possible when he took ownership of himself. This allowed him to explain which of his wife's allegations were true and which were clearly outrageous lies designed to gain sympathy for her.

This is an extreme example, yet it illustrates an important point. When our worst fears are left in the dark, they can overwhelm us and appear impossible to overcome. When we bring them into the light and face them, we can handle the result and come up with solutions. I often tell people that you don't need to know the answer to what you fear before it actually happens. You will figure it out in the moment. And despite the difficulty, we often surprise ourselves by what is possible.

Shame: I am essentially bad to have these desires

Most of us know the feeling of shame. Some of us know it more than others, especially if we were raised by a parent or guardian who used shame to control our behavior. Statements like "shame on you" often ring through our memories. One of my grandmothers often said those words, and I hated it.

Unlike fear, which is an innate emotion, shame, embarrassment and guilt are learned as we grow. Shame is often the most debilitating of these negative emotions. It is deeply ingrained in many people's psyches, and it's difficult to overcome.

So what is shame? It's the strong and often detrimental emotion that goes to the heart of a person's self-worth. Shame is the painful feeling of humiliation or distress caused by seemingly wrong or foolish behavior. ("Shame," 2017) Yet it is more than just embarrassing yourself by doing something foolish; shame attacks your sense of worth and worthiness. For example, research shows that lesbian, gay, bisexual and transgender (LGBT) youth have elevated rates of suicide, alcohol and drug abuse, and other self-destructive behaviors. Shame and pride are powerful emotions that have been historically linked to nonconformist sexual identities (McDermott, Roen, & Scourfield, 2008) like the unique sexual behaviors this book explores. Clearly, shame is a negative emotion that must be taken seriously due to the extreme consequences when it is left to fester. Mounting evidence demonstrates that the weight of shame on an individual's mental health can exacerbate cardiac problems and depress the immune system. This suggests that we should monitor our personal insecurities as much as we focus on diet, exercise, or smoking. For the sake of our hearts and bodies, we need to treat our self-image gently. (Maxmen, 2007)

Shame is a very common negative emotion in the sexual arena, whether your interests are unique or typical. Unfortunately, the field of psychotherapy often perpetuates sexual shame. The typical diagnosing therapists have been taught to use shames people who are interested in sexual-relational creativity and behavioral nonconformity. Arousing and healthy sexuality requires the very behaviors and fantasies that our sex-phobic institutions and culture want to annihilate. (Donague, 2015, p. 9) Even people with very typical sexual interests hold deep shame about their sexual desires. I once worked with a couple where the woman had deep shame about her enjoyment of anal stimulation. Even though she received her strongest orgasms from this type of sexual play and we attempted to normalize this activity for her. However, once her shame kicked in, she refused to discuss it or allow her husband of 30 years to ever engage in it again! If someone with a desire that nearly all sexual therapists would consider typical can become this shamed, just imagine the level of shame experienced by those whose desires most of society finds difficult to understand. People who feel shame suffer. Shamed people want to change, hide, or get rid of themselves. (Kashdan & Biswas-Diener, 2014, p. 83)

Our culture creates and maintains many unrealistic models about sex, one of which is the shame model. This model expects individuals to hide that they are sexual, allowing no overt or open sexual dialogue or recognition. It does not support the use of erotic capital, where one confidently leads with and utilizes their sexuality for gain and advancement. It includes sexphobic words like "whore," "pervert," and "sex addict." (Donague, 2015, p. 30) Without a doubt, when it comes to sex, shame does far more harm than good.

Embarrassment: What will others think of me?

Embarrassment is a self-conscious emotion that often shares company with guilt and shame. Because it often happens in relation to other people, embarrassment can be considered a public emotion that makes you feel exposed, awkward, and filled with regret for your alleged wrongdoing. It tells you that you failed to behave according to certain social standards, which threatens your beliefs about how others evaluate you and how you evaluate yourself. (Lamia, 2011) Other researchers have shown that embarrassment can also occur when we act in a way that is inconsistent with our personal standards. (Reivich & Shatte, 2002, p. 83) So while we are embarrassed breaching a personal value, and doing so in front of others may intensify the embarrassment, it is not a required condition. People can also be embarrassed when alone.

As mentioned earlier, our embarrassment surrounding sexual issues is one we learn, not one with which we are born. Children are not innately embarrassed by their naked bodies, genitals, or sexual responses until adults teach them to be. Children notice the uncomfortable response of the adults around them when they ask questions about sex and observe the modesty and embarrassment of those same adults. Whether people have typical or atypical sexual interests, embarrassment keeps many of them from enjoying the full expression of their sexuality.

The fact that so many women and men in our society have body image issues speaks to the level of embarrassment people have about their bodies. We are embarrassed by our sexual desires, by our lack of knowledge and experience with sex, or by a belief that we have had too many sexual experiences. The fear and shame relating to our sexuality, even when it is very typical, is extremely debilitating for many people, especially if they also struggle with self-esteem and self-image. Those with lower self-esteem are especially vulnerable to the Big Four when it comes to sexuality.

The good news is that since embarrassment is a learned response to sexuality, it can also be unlearned. I sometimes tell the story of how, at age 22, I had an hour-long, detailed conversation with my recently-divorced mother about how to perform oral sex on a man. If I could learn to be comfortable with this intimate level of discussion at a young age—with my own mother, no less—then embarrassment about sexuality can certainly be changed. Don't get me wrong, the entire experience was not without some embarrassment for both of us. However, her desire to learn and my belief that every woman, even my mother, needed this vital information got us through it. In addition, we were able to enjoy a little humor in the moment. And humor can often lessen embarrassment.

So how does someone become less embarrassed and more able to admit they are sexual beings? First, take a deep breath, let it out and admit, at least to yourself, that you feel embarrassed. Attempting to run away from the feeling only makes it worse. Also, instead of obsessing about what you are feeling, accept your imperfections. No one is perfect. And finally, stop worrying about what others think of you. Most of us exaggerate our flaws while assuming others have fewer flaws than we do. Most people don't notice the things we worry about, so learn to laugh it off and move on.

Guilt: I have done something wrong

Shame's close cousin is known as guilt. These two negative emotions often go hand-in-hand and can be difficult for many people to differentiate. However, they are very different. Shame is experienced as feeling badly about who we are. We experience guilt when we feel bad about something we did. (Aaron, 2016, p. 109) There are contrasting beliefs about whether feeling guilty is a positive or negative thing. Some people believe that guilt evolved to help us change our course of action and make amends for things we have done. Along these lines, guilt can be grouped into two categories:
   • Breaches of self-regulation, including procrastination, binge eating and drinking, failing to exercise, and overspending

- Breaches of commitment, including sexual infidelities, not spending enough time with family, and ignoring the needs of friends

When our guilt stems from situations like overeating, procrastinating, or wasting money, awareness of our breakdown in self-control can be a positive use for guilt. It can get us to stop doing the activity that is generating the guilt. If we feel guilty about having harmed others, we can apologize and try to repair the damaged relationship.

The problem is that guilt is pervasive. Researchers have found that on average, adults feel moderately guilty for 39 minutes a day. Now that's a lot of guilt! (Reivich & Shatte, 2002) Guilt is prevalent in our society as a means of controlling other people's behavior. Most of us only have to look at our family and friends to see how often guilt is used in an attempt to control us. We often hear the stereotypes of the (insert religious, ethnic, or geographic location) mother and her ability to instill guilt.

While there may be positive aspects of guilt, there are researchers who believe the opposite. Some state that "Guilt is worse than useless." Jon Connelly, PhD, believes that guilt has nothing to do with what you did or didn't do. We might think of guilt as something that improves behavior, but it often has the opposite effect. You see people with drinking problems who continue to drink due to guilt about their drinking. People put off calling a friend or family member due to their guilt for not having already called. The amount of guilt someone feels is rarely proportional to the terrible thing they have done. How is it helpful when someone who didn't remember to call a family member is guilt-ridden, yet the person who swindled multiple people out of their life savings feels no guilt at all? (Connelly, 2012)

So yes, even the experts on guilt can be confusing. I believe that while there are positive uses for guilt, it creates far more harm than good. A small amount of guilt goes a long way, so when it comes to guilt, less is more. This is especially true when it comes to sex and sexuality.

I often see this with people who are having trouble embracing their atypical sexuality because they feel guilty about not telling their partners of their desires sooner. They feel guilt for asking their partner to change the dynamics of a sexual relationship that may have started much differently than what they want now. Though the expectations for marriage have changed dramatically from 100 years ago, we still use the same language during our wedding vows (for-saking all others, 'til death do us part) that we have used for centuries. This causes people to feel guilty when they want to re-negotiate the relationship contract. Since very few people have a truly frank discussion before marriage of what their lifetime sexual expectations will be, this can be quite difficult.

I often remind people that individuals change throughout their lives and it is unrealistic to expect that your marriage or sex life will be the same at 45 as it was at 25. You shouldn't feel guilty because you have evolved. Let's face it; it's likely that your spouse has evolved as well over the years. Perhaps there is something s/he would like to disclose to you?

Putting it all together

I have no doubt you have experienced the Big Four emotions. What is uncertain is how well are you able to identify when you are feeling these emotions. Do you know when others around you are feeling them? How well do you manage them? Do you allow these emotions (your own or someone else's) to control you or overwhelm you? There is a big difference between experiencing our feelings and letting them control our behavior. Just because you feel fear, shame, embarrassment or guilt regarding atypical sexual desires doesn't mean those feelings should stop you from exploring and accepting yourself as you are.

In the 1990s, the term "emotional intelligence" or EQ became known as another area of human intelligence just as important as intellectual intelligence, or IQ. While IQ predicts an individual's capacity for logic, abstract thought, and understanding of facts, EQ is the ability to recognize one's own emotions and the emotions of others and label them accordingly. Someone with a strong EQ knows the difference between what is important to them and what's important to someone else. (Segal, 1997) While IQ is pretty much set and established by a certain age, EQ is something that a person can work on and improve. If you have a difficult time managing your emotions or the emotions of those around you, the good news is that you can improve in this area.

If you are wondering if your EQ needs some improvement, try taking this simple quiz. Fill in the following statements with *never, rarely, sometimes, frequently* or *always*. Answer the questions as quickly as possible so you are not relying on the intellectual side of your brain

1. Feeling left out or ignored troubles me. (never, rarely, sometimes, frequently, always)
2. When I have done something I'm ashamed of, I can admit it. (never, rarely, sometimes, frequently, always)
3. It upsets me when a stranger is less than friendly to me. (never, rarely, sometimes, frequently, always)
4. I can laugh at my vulnerabilities. (never, rarely, sometimes, frequently, always)
5. I beat myself up for making mistakes. (never, rarely, sometimes, frequently, always)

6. I can recognize my imperfections without feeling guilty. (never, rarely, sometimes, frequently, always)
7. When someone gets angry at me, it spoils my day. (never, rarely, sometimes, frequently, always)
8. I experience a full range of feelings every day, including sadness, anger, and fear. (never, rarely, sometimes, frequently, always)
9. My intense emotions cause me to feel out of control. (never, rarely, sometimes, frequently, always)
10. I agonize over decisions or put off decision-making. (never, rarely, sometimes, frequently, always)
11. Other people's intense emotions cause me to feel out of control. (never, rarely, sometimes, frequently, always)

If your EQ is strong, you probably answered "never" or "rarely" to the odd numbered questions and "always" or "frequently" to the even-numbered questions. (Segal, 1997, p. 21-22) Notice how quickly you took the quiz; did you pause to think about some questions? Did you go back and change answers or try to figure out what you were supposed to say to each question? Some of those types of behaviors can indicate that you were using too much intellect and not enough of your feelings. In which case, you may need some work on your emotional intelligence. If you deeply struggle with this area, you may need some additional help. I recommend Dr. Jeanne Segal's book, *Raising Your Emotional Intelligence: a Practical Guide to Help You Raise Your EQ*.

Exercises

There are many exercises to improve your ability to manage your negative emotions. I find the simple ones that people actually use to be the most effective. What good are elaborate exercises if you never try them, or do them inconsistently?

People tend to think that emotions are all in our heads. But when things are working well, both your mind and body feel emotions. Physical illnesses can start with people being unaware of how their excessively strong emotions affect their bodies. Medical professionals are starting to realize that ailments such as heart and digestive diseases have strong emotional components. Ideally, when all is working well, you are aware of your emotions in your body as well as your head.

Step One: Breathing

Breathing is underrated, especially deep, calming breaths. People tend to breathe shallowly from the chest; they often are not getting enough deep, refreshing breaths. For this exercise, you will start with one hand on your chest and the other hand on your belly. Take a series of slow, deep breaths. Both your chest and your belly should be moving and lifting. This is not the time for sucking in your gut. Slowly breathe in for a count of three to four, hold it for a count of two, then slowly breathe out for a count of five to six. The 'out' breath should be slightly longer than the 'in' breath. Be sure to breathe out fully before you breathe in again, or you risk hyperventilating. Continue this for a few minutes with slow, even, and continuous breaths. Notice how you are feeling afterwards. Are you calmer and able to think more clearly? Practice these breaths once or twice a day (more often if you are feeling strong negative emotions) as a way of calming yourself and clearing your mind.

Step Two: Noticing your emotions

During the week, notice where you feel emotion in your body, especially strong positive or negative feelings. This can be anywhere: your face, jaw or tongue; your chest, shoulders, stomach, or back. While these are the more common areas, any part of your body may experience sensation when you have an emotion. It is important to notice this, because being unaware can lead to problems like overeating, drinking too much, excessive Facebook, or other activities that numb feelings rather than help you become aware of them. Before you can learn to manage emotions, you must become aware of them. Keep a simple daily log to document what you are noticing as you become aware of where you feel your emotions in your body.

Step Three: Retrain your brain

One of the simple steps I have people adopt, especially when learning to manage fear, is to retrain your brain. Think of your brain like a computer: its output is based on the data you put in. This is very helpful if you spend a lot of time telling yourself "I can't handle it" or similar expressions. Whenever you are feeling fear and questioning your ability to handle a possible situation that might happen; tell yourself, "Whatever happens, I will figure it out." This simple statement tells your mind that you don't need to have the answer to something which may never happen. It also reminds you that when you have experienced unexpected events in the past, you have managed to handle them and devise a solution. This simple technique is also helpful if you tend to feel anxiety or panic when thinking about fearful events.

Check in: How are you doing?

Take a moment to notice what you are feeling after reading this chapter. Emotions are difficult, even for people with strong EQs, so be mindful of how this may be affecting you. If you struggle with negative emotions and want to run away from them, notice this, but be kind to yourself. Lifelong patterns do not change overnight. Remember, learning to manage your emotions is possible. You can do this!

Chapter Three

Ingrained Beliefs About Sex
Where did you learn them?

Mac sits in my office feeling frustrated and not sure what to do. He has been married for 16 years and has two children in their early teens. He is successful in his career, he and his family have a comfortable life, but he doesn't feel happy. He states that he and his wife spend what little time they have together watching their children at soccer games and school events. He misses the emotional and physical intimacy they shared earlier in their marriage. He tells me he has tried to get his wife to make their relationship more of a priority, yet she refuses, spending her time on Facebook or watching cat videos. He feels lonely and most of his sexual encounters are masturbating to porn. He states he feels guilty about that, but if he initiates sex with his wife, he gets an apathetic response. If he waits for her to initiate sex, it happens once every six months. He doesn't know what to do. He wants something different, but he's afraid of change.

I wish I could say this is an isolated case. But as we approach the end of the second decade of the twenty-first century, I hear this quite often. More and more men and women are complaining about the lack of sex or any enthusiasm for sexual variety in their relationships. There are many sources of this problem. People who take their cell phones, laptops, and tablets to bed with them or have a television in the bedroom are much less likely to be having sex with their partner than those who do not. A plethora of things in the modern world vie for our attention; unfortunately, sex stops being a priority for many of us. In addition, the beliefs many of us grew up with about sex and relationships play a powerful, yet unconscious, role. These beliefs hide under the surface and begin to play out in ways we don't notice or fully understand once we get into a stable relationship. And then we unintentionally pass them on to the next generation.

Our beliefs about sexuality and relationship styles are learned at an early age and come from many sources. For better or worse, these sources give us our first impressions of emotional and physical intimacy. This happens at a developmental stage when we lack the cognitive ability to question or understand any differently. Once we grow to adulthood, our brains can analyze these beliefs for inconsistencies and determine whether they actually work for us, yet we rarely do so.

And without ever re-examining them, we consider these beliefs to be the way it is and act accordingly. Even though we eventually get other versions of how marriage, sex and relationships can work, these early impressions affect how we behave in our own relationships decades later. Whether we grow up in a city, town, or farm the people in our communities teach us as much as our family of origin. Later on, our friends and peers share what they have learned. Furthermore, we are all affected by our educational institutions and finally, the media has a huge effect on what we believe about sex and relationships. If you spend any time reading articles in popular magazines, novels throughout history, watching television shows and movies, and especially listening to popular songs you download or hear on the radio, you will find subtle (and not-so-subtle) messages about sex and relationships.

I have heard time and again from people who end up getting married, having children, and settling into a life of mediocrity— not because they deeply wanted it, but because it was ingrained in them that this was the path they "should" take. There is nothing wrong with marriage, parenting, or the typical stable life. But when it is presented as the only successful option despite evidence to the contrary— just look at the rates of divorce and infidelity—then, as the classic line goes, "Houston, we have a problem."

In this chapter, we will examine four main areas where most of us learn our sexual and relationship beliefs: family, peers and formal education, society at large, and the media. As we go along, pay attention to your own ingrained beliefs and document them. We will finish up the chapter by giving you a chance to re-examine your beliefs and help you decide if they still apply.

Family: Where it all starts

Culture and family can socialize you into believing there are specific "healthy" ways to run your relationships, even if the ways you grew up witnessing are highly dysfunctional. (Donahue, 2015) Whether you grew up with a traditional nuclear family, extended family, or another configuration, your family of origin was your first role model for sex and relationships. Few of us learn all healthy or all dysfunctional messages; usually it's a mix of both. This makes it even more confusing to sort through the mix and understand what we want in our lives.

Since we get these messages at an age when we rarely question what we are receiving, it can make things especially difficult later on. Once we are adults, most people do not re-examine what they have been taught to see if these messages make sense or apply to their adult lives. For example, many people have heard the message "Sex is dirty, save it for marriage." If sex is so dirty, why are we saving it for the person we are supposed to love the most? Does that even make sense?

We learn whether activities like masturbation (also known as self-pleasuring) are acceptable or deeply discouraged. What many people don't realize is that all babies masturbate. This means you did too, whether you remember it or not. The question is, how did the adults caring for you react to it? Did they slap your hand and tell you it was wrong to touch yourself there? Or did they tell you that it was fine to do in private, just not in the middle of the living room in front of company? This may seem like a simple example, yet it can be symbolic of the overall messages you received and under which you still operate. Do you hide the fact that you masturbate from your spouse? Do family messages about sex keep you from letting your partner know that you masturbate? Does the disapproval you fear or have experienced from your partner in the past play a role?

I once worked with a heterosexual married couple who were a classic example of early family messages gone awry. They came in to see me after a couple years of marriage because he rarely wanted or initiated sex after they were married. Prior to getting married, each of them reported an active and satisfying sex life together. Upon examining his family of origin, it became clear that his parents showed no physical or emotional affection toward each other, even sitting in separate chairs across the room while watching TV at night. He stated he never saw his parents kiss, hold hands, or hug each other in front of him or his siblings. From a child's point of view, since there was no sexual interaction between his parents, he learned that sex was not a real part of marriage. Unfortunately for my clients, this belief was so ingrained in him, and he was unwilling to examine or talk about it, that it destroyed their marriage.

Think about the messages you learned from your family about sex and relationship dynamics. Take a piece of paper and draw a vertical line down the middle. On the left side, jot down the beliefs about sex and relationships you learned from your family. We will come back to these messages later in the chapter.

Peers and formal education: Additional sources of learning

Once we are old enough to start school, our peers and the education system have a significant impact on our beliefs about relationships and sex. Our friends bring their family's beliefs to school, as do we. Most children do not want to be different from their peers and fight to fit in. The heteronormative standards of male/female, two-person relationships are set as the norm.

Teachers and curriculums perpetuate this norm with little to no education, even in most sex education classes, about same-sex or multiple person relationships. Over the past few decades, federal and state regulations have required many school districts to enact abstinence-only sex education programs. These programs do not explain contraception or how to understand and accept young, budding sexuality. Instead, they emphasize fear of pregnancy and sexually-transmitted infections (STIs). The point of sex education should not be indoctrination into heterosexual, gender-binary, procreative-directed, or pro-marriage ideals. But in our culture, education, especially around sex, is about assimilation and not freedom or choice. The curriculum is clearly biased information masquerading as objective. (Donaghue, p. 36) There is no education about pleasure as it relates to sex. And there is no education about alternative sexual expression! Because many fetishes and kinks start at an early age, those who enjoy them started having thoughts, desires and behaviors before kindergarten, or at least by puberty. Gay, lesbian and bisexual people usually know they feel differently at a very young age. But for their own physical safety, they often need to hide who they are from those around them.

However, we are seeing more high schools demonstrate greater acceptance of sexuality. Many schools now have gay/straight alliances that give LBGTQ students a place to feel heard and safe. Schools are also fighting back against abstinence-only programs in favor of more inclusive sex education. This is a good sign. However, those of us raised a few decades ago still have old messages floating around in our heads. Think about it for a little bit. What messages from your peers and formal education are you still carrying around and living by? Did you feel you had to hide your true self from your friends and peers? Are these beliefs really working for you? Write these on your sheet of paper. We will come back to this a little later.

Society at large: What will the neighbors think?

Have you ever heard someone say, "But what will the neighbors think?" If so, you understand the power communities have over us, especially if we are dealing with unique sexual behaviors and relationships. People often allow neighbors, co-workers, and even the people in the grocery store to affect their behaviors. While in extreme cases this can have a positive effect on overall society, there are far more situations where concern about what society thinks of us is overrated.

Social control and conformity are strengthened by individual acts, like referring to certain sexual behaviors as "normal" or labeling and shaming others as "abnormal." (Donaghue, p. 9) These terms are steeped in judgment; after all, what is normal? And who decides what's normal? The ways society uses this judgment against people with unique sexual behaviors and relationship dynamics is very real. For example, if you are in a polyamorous relationship (where you have more than one committed partner), what happens if you bring your spouse and boy/girlfriend to the company holiday party? Will you get the raise and promotion you were expecting or will it go to the co-worker in a more traditional relationship? If you are involved in a BDSM (bondage and discipline, dominance/submission, sado-masochism) relationship, do you talk about the enjoyable time you had at the dungeon when your co-worker asks what you did over the weekend? Probably not! For these types of relationships, the power of societal pressure has very real consequences.

There is a definite culture war in our society when it comes to sexuality. Those who fear and hate sexuality, known as erotophobes, are attacking those who appreciate or tolerate sexuality, known as erotophiles. While erotophiles are not actively working to force erotophobes to live more sexually adventurous lives, erotophobes insist that everyone should live according to their specific values. Erotophiles who want to go to a nude beach, a strip club, a dungeon, or a swing club do not expect erotophobes to attend. Yet erotophobes are so opposed to these things that they fight to close them down so no one has the option to make these choices for themselves. (Klein, 2006)

I could write multiple chapters on society's effect on people with alternative means of sexual expression; there are many, many examples. Our culture and its institutions work against the liberation you value and need. Liberation requires examining long-held beliefs and the ways we are feeding the dominant culture. (Donaghue, 2006) After hiding for so long, subtle behavior changes become so second nature that most of those who engage in these lifestyles don't even notice. Think about the ways you have adapted what you talk about, how you dress or how you act in order to make erotophobes around you comfortable. Add these things to your sheet of paper. Do you need a second sheet? Once again, we will address this soon.

The media: The messages are everywhere

The media! What a powerful force it is, especially when it comes to sex and relationships. And in our overly consumer-driven culture, advertisers on Madison Avenue and across the country sure know how to push our buttons. While society has been affected by stories from Shakespeare to romantic books of each era, the twentieth and twenty-first centuries have taken media influence to a whole new level. When filmmaking debuted in the early twentieth century, people flocked to this new art form. Makers of early films visually engrained the cultural messages of the time about sexual mores and expectations. Fast forward to radio, television, magazines and the popular love songs of each generation. In the twenty-first century the internet accelerated the media's effect on our culture. Streaming TV, websites, social media, smartphones, tablets and all sorts of other devices constantly bombard viewers with messages about sex and relationships.

And now, we have to add social media to the equation. Social media is one of the most powerful forms of sexual socialization and education. Whether on computers or cellphones, people are extremely connected and therefore adversely affected by what they read on Facebook, Twitter, Instagram, as well as sex/dating sites such as Tinder, Grinder, (the list goes on and on). These sites affect people's sexual psyches by forming and solidifying perceptions about sex, bodies, social values and norms. The images people expose themselves to influence self-esteem, body image, as well as sexual shame and embarrassment. (Donaghue, 2015) Consider the current undertones on social media regarding slut shaming and sexual harassment;

most of which goes unreported or at best is highly under-reported. Slut shaming is the experience of labeling a woman's sexual behavior as being "out of control" when a man exhibiting the same behavior would be considered acceptable. Basically, it is the ultimate sexual double standard. Social media often gives people a way of expressing hateful, shameful, and inaccurate opinions while hiding behind their devices.

Media advertisers reinforce problematic narratives and sexist, biased presentations of "normal" sexuality. Genders are always clearly male or female and relationships are nearly always heterosexual, monogamous, and nuclear-family centered. Since same-sex marriage became legal across the country, a few gay and lesbian couples now appear in ads, yet there are no representations of polyamory, open marriages, sex-for-fun-only relationships or alternative family configurations. (Donaghue, 2015) As humans, we tend to look for ourselves in the images we see. Most advertising is clearly directed at Caucasian, heterosexual, legally-married couples. So what are the rest of us supposed to see and subconsciously ingest? For many sexual minorities, the message is that you are different, unwelcome, and not important enough to portray in popular culture. Think about this for a few minutes. What messages have you internalized about being different in a culture that states that we value individuality, yet obviously promotes conformity? Add these to your sheet of paper.

Examining old beliefs: Do they still apply to you now?

Luckily for me, I was the type of teenager to question almost everything. This trait served me well as I questioned the beliefs I had been raised with and stopped living by the ones that did not work for me. As I look around, I realize that many others didn't do the same.

Let's go back to the beliefs about sex and relationships we discussed in this chapter and I have asked you to notice and write down.

Read them over again. Are there ones on the list that still work in your sexual life? If so, put a star next to them on the far-left side.

Now, look at the beliefs on your list that no longer apply to your adult self. On the right side, start writing new beliefs to replace them. You may already have been living different beliefs, yet have not embraced them and fully acknowledged them to yourself. This exercise gives you a chance to see them in black and white, which can be very powerful for the subconscious part of your brain. Start taking ownership of what you now want to believe about sex and relationships as you move forward.

Check in: How are you doing?

Challenging long-held beliefs, especially those from family, can feel like a threat to the status quo or even a betrayal to those who you love. Think about and identify the people in your life who will be threatened if you make changes to your sexual and relationship dynamics.

Chapter Four

The War on Men's Sexuality
The forces trying to control you

Unless you have been living in a cave, you have heard the story of Tiger Woods. Famous, rich, attractive, successful athlete married to a beautiful blond supermodel. He apparently had it all. What was wrong with him, sneaking around with multiple other women? Clearly, he had a problem! Tiger Woods is one of the more famous causalities of the current war on sexuality.

What most people don't know is that when he was a teenager, Tiger was a tall, skinny nerd with thick glasses; golf was the focus of his life. He wasn't exactly a chick magnet. However, once he became famous, it is believed those who were sculpting his image got him corrective eye surgery, buffed up his muscles, improved his wardrobe and married him off to a beautiful model to create the perfect celebrity. Now that Tiger was attractive, successful and very rich, women were throwing themselves at him. This was something he was not prepared for. While it is easy to demonize and judge him, let's face it—how many of us could have fought off that level of temptation?

For centuries, part of the job of a civilized society was to control the people living in that society to keep peace and prevent chaos. While this can have many positive aspects, the need for control can become problematic, especially when it comes to the unique sexual behaviors of consenting adults. Societies throughout history kept strong control over women's sexuality, and women who ventured outside expectations paid a hefty price. Even now, think about the many names we call women who openly enjoy their sexuality: slut, whore, tramp, jezebel, fallen woman, skank…the list goes on and on. There were not an equal number of negative messages for men who enjoy their sexuality until recently. Over the past few decades, men's sexuality has come under fire and a new, false theory of sex and pornography has become the new means by which society, religion, politics, and even the psychotherapy world control men sexually. What is the new term? *Sex Addict!* Those who have been fueling this façade have done an excellent job convincing the masses that this actually is a legitimate diagnosis when all credible research finds the opposite.

This false theory of sex and porn addiction is a huge problem, and many men are being demonized over it. However that is not the only factor in this war on men's sexuality. There is a battle between men and women that I like to call the Gender War as well as conservative religious and political forces that must be addressed to understand the full scope of the problem.

In this chapter, we will examine the many forces that are working to control everyone's sexuality, especially men. We will look at the false theory of sex and porn addiction and how religion, politics, and the Gender War are out to control us all. While people who enjoy alternative means of sexual expression have the most to lose, even those with more typical sexuality are at risk. This is important because if the forces out to control sexuality are successful, all of us lose.

Sex and porn addiction: A flawed theory becomes an alleged epidemic

The sexual openness of the 1960s and 70s lead into the sexually-repressed 80s and 90s. Historically, the pendulum of societal norms swings back and forth. There are few more drastic examples of such a quick shift of societal norms than the sexual views between these time frames. The second time frame, the 1980s and 90s, bore much of the sexual repression that we still see in evidence today. These decades gave birth to the Religious Right, the anti-porn movement, and the creation of a theory called "sex addiction." We have Patrick Carnes to thank for this rigid and flawed theory. The whole idea of sex addiction is borne out of a moralistic ideology masquerading as science. It is a concept that serves no other purpose than to relegate sexual expression to a shameful act except within the extremely narrow and myopic scope of a monogamous, heterosexual marriage. What about sexual diversity? Interest in unique forms of sex or high-frequency sexual expression? Open relationships and non-monogamy? Advocates of sex addiction would label these the uncontrollable acts of a sexually pathological individual who needs to be cured. (Taverner, 2008, p. 11) While there are certainly cases where sexual behavior can become problematic or out of control, they are very different from what the sex addiction theory would have people believe.

Those in the sex addiction movement state that they have scientific proof of their flawed theory. However, when carefully examined, the field of sex addiction is a belief system, not a scientific or medical school of thought. The cult of sex addiction is driven by charismatic and convincing leaders who espouse sensationalist and reactive views of sexuality based on their own experiences, conviction, and religious faith, NOT on science or valid research. (Ley, 2012, p. 211) If you have ever researched the cost of a sex addiction treatment facility, you will quickly see that it is a big business. A hugely profitable business that doesn't want people questioning their beliefs.

Much of the psychotherapy world has been fooled by this scientifically-flawed concept. The American Association of Sexuality Educators, Counselors and Therapists (AASECT), which is considered the premier professional organization for sexuality professionals, struggled with whether they agree or disagree with the concept of sex addiction for decades. Even though this discussion started over 30 years ago, it took until 2017 for AASECT to finally create a position statement *condemning* the concept of sex addiction. That indicates a high level of belief in this flawed concept. When professionals who spend their lives researching and studying the vast variety of human sexuality have a difficult time labeling something as a flawed theory, how is the general public supposed to know better?

For those who explore alternative means of sexual expression, this issue is very important, because as you start to embrace your true self and express it more fully, there are many people who will want to label you a sex addict. Do not believe them. If you are wondering if you might have a sincere problem controlling your sexual behavior, there are several excellent books to use as resources. *The Myth of Sex Addiction* by David Ley and *America's War on Sex* by Marty Klein are two of the best books on the subject.

Religion and politics: Powerhouses of control

Many people grow up with strong religious beliefs that add positive aspects to their lives. But while not all religions have rigid views on human sexuality, conservative religions have twisted the gift of sexuality into something for people to fear. These same religions have contributed to our cultural ignorance surrounding Eros, sacred sexuality, and the human body. Some people turn to conservative religion for answers in their quest for meaning and once there, they are promised a "happily ever after" if they wait for sex until marriage or marry a person of their own faith. However, they usually discover that the rules fail to deliver. (Schermer Sellers, 2017)

Growing up in religious, sexually-repressed households that teach abstinence only-sex education leaves people ill-prepared for difficulties in their sex lives after marriage. They may also find they have no one in their conservative religious community to turn to for answers. And since often they have been taught not to trust the secular community, those who *do* have the answers are considered suspect.

For those who were raised in conservative religious communities, the Big Four feelings of fear, shame, guilt and embarrassment are welded upon the psyches of the faithful, especially when it comes to sex. And for those who enjoy alternative means of sexual expression, the price is especially high. I see individuals struggling because they feel they must choose between their religious faith and their sexuality. What a difficult choice!

Some people wonder what politics have to do with sex. As someone who spent 14 years working in clinics that provided contraceptive and abortion care, I can tell you that the personal is political. Politics has its own agenda when it comes to controlling sexuality in general and alternative sexuality specifically. Politics also colludes with organized religion. After all, America's religiously themed anti-sex program couldn't succeed without active, enthusiastic government participation. Why would federal and state governments care enough to join religion in repressing sexuality? While there are a variety of reasons, it is due primarily to the twin evils of politics, money and power, along with something rarely found in government—personal belief. People who believe their religion instructs them that everyone should live as they do have gotten elected to various levels of government. They inject their religious beliefs into laws and regulations we all have to adhere to. (Klein, 2006) So much for the separation of church and state!

After the 2016 presidential election, the influence of religion and politics on alternative sexuality can seem especially frightening. I have spent many hours in my office with my alternative sexuality clients, calming their very real fears. What I tell them, in essence, is to remember that it is often darkest before the dawn. There are many people and organizations educating and advocating for a better world for those who express their sexuality differently. The National Coalition for Sexual Freedom (NCSF) is one of many organizations fighting for the rights of sexual minorities. Be aware of the influences of both organized religions and political forces. Just because they are strong doesn't mean they will win.

The Gender War: Why are we fighting each other?

When it comes to sexuality, there has been a war between the genders for a long time. It is a war that is counterproductive in that it hurts both sides; yet it is one that our upbringing and society strongly promote. Think back to your teen years. Whether in your family or the families of friends and neighbors, most of us have seen the beginning of this battle. As teens enter puberty and begin to consider dating, what is the dominant message?

Many girls are told to think about their reputation, a regulation that strives to keep them from becoming sexually active. For many boys, the message is the opposite—sow your wild oats and prove what a stud you are. Girls are taught to withhold sex, while boys are taught to push to get as much as possible. Girls are taught to clamp down on any sexual feelings from a young age and wait until they are in a serious relationship before "giving in." Once in a marriage or serious relationship, they are supposed to magically flip the switch and be interested in sex. For many of the women I treat for low sexual desire in marriage, these early mixed messages play a crucial role.

I am starting to see many more encouraging scenarios where parents are instructing their boys about sexual respect, like "No means no," and encouraging their girls to think about sex as being fun in addition to messages about how to best protect themselves. However, those who were teenagers 20, 30, or 40 years ago did not grow up learning that message. For many people in mid-life, it is still operating today like an old edition of Windows 3.0.

Our society teaches us that men and women are so different from each other that of course there will be trouble between the genders. In reality, we have far more in common. All embryos are exactly the same for the first few weeks of development except for whether they have an extra X or a Y chromosome.

Once we develop beyond the embryonic stage, there are basically two major gender differences. First is the amount of the sex hormones—testosterone, estrogen, and progesterone—we each have in our systems. Although both genders have all three hormones, levels vary between individuals, so there are a wide range of differences between individual men and individual women. These hormones are powerful chemicals, so make no mistake, they certainly affect us.

The second difference is the way each gender is raised in their family and society. Since the rules for men and women are often very different, this can clearly affect individual people differently. To say that men are one way, and women are another way is an inaccurate generalization. While some personality traits are found more often in men or women, all of them can be found in both genders.

I realize this may seem like a simplistic description of the many forces that create real and imagined differences between the genders.

This topic could be its own book. At some point, both sides must realize that the price for this battle is too high. We have more to gain from putting aside our egos and working towards a truce.

So how do we get past all the fighting and come to neutral ground between the genders when it comes to sexuality? First, we have to admit that we have been taught to battle each other. It can be very difficult to put down indoctrinated beliefs. Second, we need to realize that both men and women really want the same things: to be loved, accepted, feel connected, enjoy pleasure, and feel appreciated. As individuals, we may have learned different ways to achieve these things; as partners, we may need to listen more closely to each other in order to learn how we both get our needs met.

Don: The average "sex/porn addict"

Multiple men in my practice start by telling me that they are "sex addicts" and need help with their problem. There are usually several common factors for these men, so we will call the average sex/porn addict "Don" for simplification.

When Don comes into my office, his female partner has usually diagnosed him as a sex addict after seeing an episode of Dr. Phil or a similar show. Don often has a history of limited or negative messages about sex from his family of origin. This doesn't give him much knowledge on the subject, and most of the knowledge he has is rather skewed. Don usually has a dysfunctional sexual relationship with his partner, who still operates under the negative and controlling messages about sex she grew up with. She is very rigid and controlled about their sexual behaviors or has decided she no longer wants sex at all. She also thinks that because she no longer wants sex, Don should feel the same. Basically, she wants to hold him as a sexual hostage.

Both men and women are visually stimulated to sexual arousal. Research generally indicates that men are more visual; with women, it depends on the context in which images are presented. Regardless, Don uses sexual imagery (also known as porn) to mentally stimulate himself when he masturbates. Since he does not want to cheat on his spouse, this is often his only sexual outlet. But now, Don is further punished by being told he is a sex/porn addict for engaging in any self-pleasuring behavior. He feels large amounts of shame, guilt and embarrassment. No wonder Don is so easily manipulated by the sex addiction movement.

If someone spends many hours a day watching football, binge-watching their favorite TV series, or interacting on Facebook, we deem them "normal." If they watch an hour of porn in that same day, they must have an addiction. For those who have sexual interests they fear divulging to their partner, watching those images in porn may be their only outlet.

Do not misunderstand. There are people who spend 16 hours a day watching porn rather than engage with their partners, spend their rent money on sex workers, or spend hours searching online for random hookups, all of which affect their work, families, relationships, and personal lives. For these people, their sexuality has gotten out of control and they *do* need professional help.

However, the majority of people who have been sent to me for help with sex addiction do not meet this criterion. Most of these men and women need better education about sexuality, help sorting out their own desires and emotions, and couples counseling to help with the mismatch in sexual desires with their partners.

How do these forces control you?

The sex addiction movement, conservative religion, politics, and the gender war are woven into the fabric of our current society. And as we explored in the last chapter, our culture and society have a huge effect on our beliefs and behaviors so whether you realize it or not, these aspects probably effect you as well.

Think about how often people talk about someone being a sex addict as if they understand the concept of what they are saying. Notice, on whatever news source you use, how politics work to control sexuality. Contraceptive coverage in insurance is a controversial issue, yet erectile dysfunction medications for men are easily covered. And what about the ongoing battle between men and women? The societal belief that is still perpetuated is the myth that good girls don't really want sex and men want it all the time. Clearly this is not true, since half the heterosexual couples coming into sex therapy for low sexual desire are because the man no longer desires sex. And imagine the shame of the man who has to admit to a therapist that he doesn't fit the societal belief that all men want sex all the time.

Once you start noticing the effects of these issues in our culture and society, little by little they will begin to ring out loud and clear. Since we all grow up with these cultural messages from a young age, we often don't even notice them later on. When you do begin to notice them, you will have a difficult time seeing anything else.

Exercises

For the next week, I want you to keep a journal listing all the examples in both your immediate and larger world of the various forces we have talked about in this chapter. Notice the subtle effects of these forces and how they attempt to control your sexuality. Notice how the media, friends, family and your partner subtly use the false theory of sex/porn addiction or religion, politics and the gender war to control you or others around you. Pay extra attention to ways in which you modify your own behavior due to these forces. Write down what you notice.

Check in: How are you doing?

Lifting the veil on the multiple forces out to control your sexuality (as well as the sexuality of others) can bring up a lot of emotions. It can feel like a hopeless uphill battle. Notice the feelings, but do not give in to them. We still have some distance to go. These four chapters were designed to give you an understanding of the history of our ingrained beliefs about sex so you have a solid foundation for the work ahead. The next few chapters will give you information to help you grow before we get to the final, more challenging chapters.

Chapter Five

Permission to Explore
From my permission to your own

"Dr. Rhoda, I have to tell you something, but I am afraid you are going to think I am weird." I have heard this statement many times. And while I do my best to assure everyone who says this that they are unlikely to shock me, they usually think their issue is the worst. Sometimes they wonder if I can cure their fetish or will tell them to abstain from their perceived weird sexual behaviors. They are surprised when that is very rarely what I say.

As someone who specializes in alternative sexuality, I have often found myself in the position of giving permission. People who come to work with me are looking for more than answers, they are looking for permission. Permission to know that they are OK for thinking differently, being different, and permission to explore what some of those differences mean. They have been holding themselves back for many years, fearing what people might think or say. Keeping these desires in the dark only breeds fear, lack of confidence, and hurts people's ability to be objective in their judgment. Together, my clients and I bring these desires into the light so together we can examine them objectively.

The majority of alternative sexual behaviors people present to me, including the ones we are talking about in this book, are well within the acceptable range of human sexual expression. Yes, many of them are rather unique and atypical from what you see in society or the media. This does not make these alternative sexualities "weird," and it certainly doesn't make them wrong. However, because there are times when desires are **not** okay (non-consensual or harmful to others, for example), we need to discuss when permission is granted and when it is denied to have a clear understanding of what is acceptable.

In this chapter, we will focus most of our attention on when permission to explore is granted and encouraged and when it is not. We will look at how you can take my permission and learn to grow it into your own. We will also help assess if you are ready for the changes you are craving and about to explore.

Earlier in my career, I worked at a treatment center for sexual offenders. Most of these men and women were not true pedophiles in that they were not sexually aroused by children. They were people whose sexual thoughts and fantasies had gotten out of control. They didn't have anyone to help them realize their judgement was off. Those who fit these criteria and for whom permission to explore is denied should consider seeking professional help for dangerous desires. Dangerous desires include having sex with someone who is passed out from alcohol or drugs or drugging someone's drink so you can have sex with them.

Permission: When it is granted

In chapters six and seven, we will go into much more detail about common alternative sexual behaviors I see and help people accept. This is not an exhaustive list; this would be a very long book if it were. But the central question is, how does one know when permission to explore alternative and unique means of sexual expression is given? The big issues to understand here are intent and consent.

When I am deciding whether to give someone I am working with permission to explore their desires, I am thinking about two very important issues. I am looking for both intent and consent in what they want and how they desire to engage in their unique behaviors.

First, let's consider intent. Here are a few of the things I ask my clients to consider: What do you want to get out of this experience? Is there a desire for mutual pleasure or is it one-sided? Are you willing to educate your partner about your unique desires or do you want to exert pressure and control to get your partner to engage?

This leads into the second issue, consent. Is your partner truly willing to explore or are you attempting to slip your desire under the radar and hope s/he doesn't notice? Are you attempting to use an unhealthy power advantage to get someone to agree? And a very important area to consider: is your partner a consenting adult, or someone underage?

Let me give you a couple examples to clarify what we are talking about. Beth and Danny came to see me to learn how to open up their marriage. She had been thinking about this and researching it as well as dropping hints to Danny for months. It finally came to a head when she told him she had given in to a sexual liaison with a co-worker.

Once we finished working through the feelings of hurt and betrayal regarding the indiscretion, we could start exploring each partner's feelings around wanting more than traditional marriage was giving them. Their intent was to keep what was good and strong about their marriage. We explored how they could begin this new phase of their marriage and sex life together.

The second example is a bit more unusual. Since my doctoral dissertation on adult babies and diaper fetishes, I have become one of the experts in the psychotherapy world on the subject. This has given me the experience of working with people who express their sexuality and personality in this way. In the vast majority of cases, the people I see fit the definition of positive intent and consent. Their intent is for their partner to understand what makes their fetish important and how they can negotiate a way for them both to consent and allow each other to get their needs met. While they often fear disclosing it, once they do, we begin working on how to use it in a positive manner.

Take, for example, John and Amy. They had been married for eight years and had two young children. For many years, John struggled with wanting to wear diapers as part of sex play. He hid it from Amy, hoping the desires would go away. Eventually he realized he had to tell her about his secret desires. The uniqueness of this fetish meant they had to have a lot of in-depth conversations in order for her to understand.

People confuse a diaper fetish with pedophilia, which it is not. John did not want to have sex with children. He wanted to wear a diaper and have his very adult wife engage with him sexually. John realized it would be difficult to slip his fetish under the radar, so he was forced to be vulnerable and have some difficult conversations. I have heard examples of someone springing out of the bathroom in a diaper, hoping to avoid a difficult conversation and that their partner would be OK with it. Rarely is that the case. Most of the time in situations like this, there are a lot of conversations before there is actual engagement. This is usually also a very privately-kept fetish. There are exceptions to this example, which we will explore in the next section.

Permission: When it is denied

When people think about the negative aspects of sexuality, intent to harm or someone taking what they want without consent often comes to mind. There is a reason that the DSM 5 (Diagnostic and Statistical Manual for Mental Disorders, fifth edition) lists disorders that are not only serious issues in therapy, but illegal, under "Paraphilic Disorders." These issues include voyeuristic disorder, where someone receives sexual arousal from observing an unsuspecting person who is naked or involved in a sexual act. Exhibitionistic disorders involve receiving sexual arousal from exposing one's genitals to an unsuspecting person in public. People with frotteuristic disorders are aroused by sexually touching or rubbing against a non-consenting person. Usually this is done in a crowded train, bus, or other enclosed space so the perpetrator can slip away in the crowd. And finally, adults with pedophilic disorder are aroused by sexual interaction with pre-pubescent children. (*DSM 5*, 2013)

These are the obvious and extreme examples of when permission to explore one's unique sexual desires is clearly denied. However, there are some less-obvious examples I want to share with you to give you a full understanding of what I have seen.

I once had a client who was seeking help starting an open relationship. He was married and they had always had a traditional, monogamous agreement. He wanted to explore having sex with other partners. In a true open relationship, both partners consent to the agreement and the intent is for both to enjoy it. Unfortunately, my client didn't want to tell his wife or give her the option of being sexual with other people. His *intent* was to slip this under her radar without getting her *consent*. I had to tell him that what he was proposing was not an open relationship, but adultery.

Let's go back to another example from the adult baby/diaper fetish world where permission would be denied. If someone wanted to go to a public place like a shopping mall in a diaper and onesie and suck on a pacifier while being pushed around in a larger stroller, this type of behavior would be discouraged. It is not just because it is strange to see an adult in this manner. It is because the *intent* is to shock and pull other people into this person's "scene" without their *consent.*

Thankfully, I have experienced far more times where I give permission and encourage exploration than the opposite.

How to grow your inner permission

When I am working with someone and give them permission to explore, I tend to see it like a set of training wheels. My permission is designed to get them started: eventually they need to learn to ride on their own without support. How long the training wheels stay on varies from person to person. Some clients learn to ride independently very quickly while others need more time and guidance. There is no right or wrong amount of time for this to happen. Giving you permission to explore is designed to encourage you to expand your horizons and step out of your usual comfort zone. I will give you an example later in this chapter when we talk about how David and Mac dealt with this exact issue in very different ways.

So how do you learn to grow your inner permission? A large part of it has to do with your level of self-confidence. Confidence is different than being selfish and narcissistic. It means you can examine your own desires and balance them against the needs and wants of those around you. When someone continually puts their own needs ahead of everyone else's, we have to question the intent. Allowing others to put their wants ahead of yours is not a healthy balance either. It is important to learn how to negotiate and balance the needs of everyone involved in a relationship. Sometimes each half of a couple has changed so drastically over the years that finding common ground is no longer possible. We will explore this more in Chapter 10 when we talk about examining tough choices.

Here are some steps to begin improving your confidence and your ability to create and nurture your inner permission system.

1. Put your best foot forward: If you are not doing so already, be sure to engage in good grooming and dress nicely so you can send the best version of yourself into the world. When you present confidently, your mind will begin to believe it.

2. Stop negative thoughts: We all have too much negative self-talk. If you are telling yourself "My desires are weird," or "I shouldn't want/need this," you need to create new, less harsh thoughts to replace them.

3. Think and act positively: Not only do you need to replace negative thoughts with positive one, but you must act in a positive manner. When you change to more positive actions, you change yourself one step at a time.

4. Be willing to take risks: Before you take risks, you need to be prepared. Increase your knowledge of the area you want to explore before you dive in. Have some idea of what to expect.

5. Avoid people who treat you badly: It is difficult to be confident in yourself and your decisions if those around you continually put you down. If people who do this are unwilling to see how badly they are treating you or are unwilling to change, you may need to surround yourself with more positive people.

We will go into greater depth about this when we get to the exercises near the end of the chapter.

David and Mac: Growing with permission vs. remaining stuck

David and Mac are good examples of two ways I see people handle the situation when I give them permission to explore. You may remember, we talked about David at the beginning of Chapter One and Mac as we started Chapter Three.

David was terrified what might happen once his wife learned of his BDSM desires. His wife was a very traditional woman and for years, he had always given in to her way of operating in their marriage and sex life. He believed, correctly, that she would not want to engage in the types of sexual behaviors he wanted to explore. He didn't want to push her into doing things with less than mutual enthusiasm. Getting his newly-understood needs met required David to open the marriage and have an additional partner who wanted a BDSM relationship. He also needed to get his wife's knowledge and consent.

To be honest, this was not an easy process. It certainly took some time. But once David and his wife could agree upon what each of them needed to make it work, he was off and running. As we will disclose further in Chapters Nine and Eleven, eventually he, his wife, and his new sexual submissive were able to negotiate a polyamorous relationship that worked for the three of them.

Mac was unhappy and unfulfilled and wanted something that would give him the excitement and connection he wanted from his wife, yet she refused to discuss anything different or change her behaviors. We spent several sessions exploring his feelings and discussing possible options as well as their pros and cons. As we got to the point of granting permission to explore these possibilities, Mac froze. The fear of change was so strong that he was, at the time, unable to move forward. He cancelled his next appointment and despite further encouragement, was unable to continue. Sometimes this happens. The fear people internalize can be very strong. Some people are never able to overcome it; others just need more time.

Beyond permission: Are you really ready for this kind of change?

Now that you have been given permission to explore and are learning how to grow it within yourself, it is time to begin considering the ultimate question. *Are you really ready for this kind of change?* You do not need to answer the question at this very moment. However, it is time to begin to ponder it. Realize that as you think honestly about making changes in your sex life, your negative emotions may start to surface. This can be a good time to work on managing these emotions so they do not rule your decisions. Look back at the exercises from Chapter Two to help you remain strong. As we move further through the book, you'll find information that will help you answer this question more fully so you can make an informed decision.

I feel it is important to slowly start the process of considering if this is the best path for you to explore. The exploration is the easy part. We will get to decisions later. Right now, as you work on building your confidence and knowledge, allow yourself to dream and imagine the possibilities. You must give yourself permission to dream before you figure out how to make those dreams reality.

Exercises

Giving yourself permission to explore and increasing your self-confidence are changes created at the brain level that impact every facet of your life. We can use the power of our brains to change and improve instead of passively falling prey to our negative self-talk. Our brains are constantly renewing themselves, so using this natural tendency to promote positive thinking and reduce negative thinking can have a dramatic impact on how we live our lives. This can be done in three steps:

1. Pause and notice: Stop and listen to your self-talk habit. The first step is self-awareness. Since these thoughts are ingrained, we have to slow down our thinking in order to be aware that we are engaging in negative self-talk. Here's a good exercise for becoming aware: What do you tell yourself when you make a mistake like dropping and breaking a glass on your kitchen floor? Do you say things like "I am so stupid/clumsy/bad?" If so, ask yourself if would you say the same thing to a guest in your home if they dropped and broke the same glass. I think not. Learn to be as nice to yourself as you would to a guest in your home.

2. Stand up to yourself for yourself: Once you notice the negative things you say to yourself, you must protect yourself from negative self-talk. Don't allow yourself to talk to yourself that way. Practice changing these statements to a kinder, gentler version. If you break a glass accidently and say "I am so stupid," stop and replace it with something like, "No worries. It was an accident, it can be cleaned up." After all, isn't that what you would tell your guest? This type of practice will begin to change your brain's neurological pathways.

3. Practice what is working: As you begin to substitute positive messages for negative messages, your confidence will start to grow. Encourage yourself to practice these efforts. I like to think of it as creating new roads in your brain for automatic thoughts. Building new roads is tough when the existing negative freeways are well-traveled. But because the gift of neuroplasticity makes you capable of creating new, better roads, the old freeways grow cracked and full of weeds once they are less traveled. (Onofrey, 2017)

Check in: How are you doing?

Are you ready to move forward? Hopefully, at this point in the process you are managing your negative emotions so they are not overwhelming. The desired effect is that negative emotions are lessening, or at least manageable, and the excitement is beginning to grow. Over the next three chapters we will educate you about BDSM, fetishes, kinks, and open relationships such as swinging and polyamory. We will look at the pros and cons of each so you can feel informed and prepared for the final four chapters of the book.

Chapter Six

Exploration

The many faces of different. Come to the fun side.
We have cookies.

You may have heard the saying "Come to the Dark Side. We have cookies." It makes me smile and giggle whenever I hear it. As I was starting this chapter, it didn't seem quite appropriate to refer to this as the dark side. Many people who engage in BDSM, fetishes, and kinks do so because they enjoy it and are having fun. Sexual behavior should be fun! As humans, we engage in sex for procreation only a few times in our lives. Relational sex, which is the aspect of feeling connected to another human being, is also a strong reason for many to be sexual.

However, there is value in sex just because it's fun. This tends to be the reason most people choose to be sexual, with much greater frequency, over their lifespan. Of course, there are many reasons to engage in sex: as a coping mechanism, to relieve boredom or stress, to reduce horniness, or even to improve a bad mood. (Donaghue, 2015) Yet having sex for fun can be one of the best reasons.

When people come to see me to help them express their alternative sexuality, they usually already know exactly what they want. They may have been holding back from fully expressing these desires for many years. However, sometimes people come in knowing they need something different, but have not even given themselves permission to explore the options available to them. They just know there must be *something* more.

In this chapter, I will give you some basic information about BDSM, fetishes, kinks, and sexual orientation. Up until recently, the definition of sexual orientation was thought to be as simple as straight, gay or bisexual. Current research in the field of sexology is beginning to show that it may be much broader than the gender of the person or persons with whom you desire to be sexual. I will help you learn more about area(s) that appeal to you and provide exercises filled with resources for further self-research.

BDSM: Much more than 50 Shades

Until recently, BDSM—bondage and discipline, dominance and submission, sadomasochism—was a little-known area on the fringes of sexuality. While the *50 Shades of Grey* books and films have many people talking about BDSM, it is far from something new. Most of those in the BDSM community as well as sexuality professionals cringe at the 50 Shades books and films. As a means to expand knowledge and awareness of BDSM, the series was a huge success. However, the series fails at educating people how to perform BDSM behaviors safely and consensually. The inaccurate manner in which BDSM activities are portrayed in *50 Shades of Grey* and its sequels leaves people with dangerous ideas about how to experiment with their partner.

Knowledge about how to engage in such behaviors safely is important. For example, improper use of rope or other restraints can cut off circulation or cause nerve damage. It is imperative to learn proper technique. The same is true with spanking, flogging, or other types of impact play. Technique is critical to insure you are inflicting sensation and pain in a way that doesn't cause unnecessary bodily damage. You also need to understand the mental and physical aspects of how to slowly build the intensity of a scene as well as how to perform "aftercare."

Giving you best practices for BDSM play is really beyond the scope of this book. Many others have spent years perfecting their craft and creating books, websites, and blogs in order to share their knowledge. If you are interested in engaging in BDSM behaviors, be sure to use the resources at the end of the chapter to fully educate yourself before jumping into the deep end of the pool.

These unique sexual behaviors go way back in time and probably have always been a part of human sexuality. The "S" in the term S&M, or sadomasochism, comes from the Marquis de Sade, a French aristocrat and writer who lived in the late 1700s and early 1800s. He was a sadist who deeply enjoyed inflicting pain on consenting and non-consenting partners. The "M," masochism, comes from a writer in the 1800s named Leopold von Sacher-Masoch who was known to enjoy receiving pain in his sexual interactions.

Because BDSM covers a broad range of behaviors, it can be challenging to give you a clear understanding of them. When first educating people, I like to say that BDSM can go from mild to very wild. Technically, couples who buy the furry pink handcuffs, blindfold, and little paddle at the local sex shop to spice up their lives are engaging in BDSM activities. And yet they are far removed from those who consider themselves educated members of the BDSM community.

At its core, BDSM is about expanding levels of physical and mental sensations. The body's five senses are either limited or increased by practitioners. While physical sensations of pain and pleasure are obvious, the mental aspect of erotic power exchange is also part of BDSM. To the outsider, this can appear subtle, but for those enjoying the mental aspects of power exchange, it is significant. Erotic power exchange can range from blindfolding and restraining a partner during sex play to some form of sexual or even non-sexual servitude from the submissive partner. It can be as simple as whispering in the other's ear "I own your body for the next hour."

While some may see the behaviors as aligning with abuse, within consensual BDSM, there is a clear difference. People who engage in BDSM have explicit codes of conduct. Within the community you will hear terms like "safe, sane, and consensual" as well as "RACK: risk, aware, consensual, kink." These describe how to go about these activities in a manner that maintains healthy emotional and physical safety.

Before starting to "play," those who engage usually have in-depth discussions, often involving written contracts and inventories, that include what each side desires from the "scene," firm limits to avoid, and what areas are flexible and could be pushed in the moment. I often say that if everyone engaged in this level of communication before having sex, we would see a lot fewer problems in people's sex lives.

People who practice BDSM use roles to indicate the power differential in their exchanges. While most people stay consistent as one type of partner, some people refer to themselves as a "switch," meaning that they engage in either role, depending on their mood or the situation. In all of these roles, one partner appears to be in control and one appears to submit to that control. However, the more powerful partner does not have ultimate control over their activity. Instead, the partner who chooses to submit controls the scene, because they can stop it at any time by using a "safe word."

While people use many types of safe words, I recommend something simple that I call the Stop Light. In the heat of the moment, you do not want a word you cannot remember or one that can be misinterpreted. The Stop Light approach is simple. If either side asks if everything is "green," it means that things are good; continue to proceed. "Yellow" is for caution, which can mean either one partner needs a break or that something, such as a restraint, needs to be adjusted before the scene can continue. And just like a stoplight, "Red" means everything stops now. Only use "Red" if you are truly finished, because after it's called, the scene is done for the night.

Let's go back to the different roles. There are various levels that relate to intensity, level of involvement between the participants, and the amount of power exchanged. Either gender can play either role. First, you have a Top or a bottom. The Top is the person who controls the scene and inflicts the various sensations. The bottom is the one submitting to the scene. When people are using the term Top or bottom, this is usually a more casual type of arrangement; the roles are dropped at the end of the scene.

Next, you have Dominant/Domme and submissive roles. The Dominant/Domme is also the one in control, but there is often more commitment to the relationship. The term Dominant is often used for a male partner, while the term Domme may be used for a female partner. The submissive is giving up control for the scene. Sometimes, this arrangement can extend outside of the immediate scene to non-sexual aspects of the relationship.

Finally, you have Master/Mistress or slave. This is the highest level of the power exchange roles. In this type of arrangement, the Master/Mistress is seen as "owning" the slave. The slave chooses to submit most of their control and defers to his or her Master's/Mistress's wishes. For both the Dominant/submissive and Master/slave roles, the submissive/slave may wear a collar as a sign of their devotion and of being owned.

As you may have noticed, the Top, Dominant/Domme, and Master/Mistress roles are always capitalized while the terms bottom, submissive and slave are lowercased. This is done as a way of showing respect. For each side, showing respect is very important in this community.

If BDSM play interests you, I strongly advise you to do a great deal of research and learn as much as possible before engaging in it. You need to know the rules, expectations, and how to keep yourself and your partner safe. Unfortunately, I have worked with a couple of young, eager female submissives who met someone claiming to be an experienced Dominant who was, in reality, just a predator who beat and raped them. I tell you this not to frighten you, but to remind you to be aware—it is your responsibility to protect yourself.

Fetishes: When things themselves become exciting

In Chapter One, we met Josh, who had a shoe and foot fetish. By definition, a fetish is when an individual is intensely sexually aroused by specific objects or non-genital body parts. For some unknown reason, most people who enjoy fetishes are men. Research shows that the percentage of women who have a fetish varies. While there are many theories on the difference between the genders, the exact reasons are unknown. Many in the field of sexology believe the number of women with some level of fetish may be higher than reported. In my professional opinion, there is a level of sexism at play here, as many of the traditional male researchers have difficulty imagining women enjoying sexual fetishes.

Most people who have a fetish (or multiple fetishes) are capable of being sexually aroused without the fetish item. In the cases where the fetish item is always necessary, sex therapy is usually warranted to expand their interests to sexual behavior both with and without the fetish item. This is because the partner of someone with a fetish feels inconsequential and unimportant if the fetish item is always necessary.

The majority of the time, a fetish is a harmless quirk and way to express one's sexuality. The problem is that fetish items or behaviors can seem rather strange to a partner who has never been educated about their partner's unique sexual interest. Many people with fetishes hold deep shame and embarrassment: due to fear of rejection, hiding these desires isn't unusual.

Fetishes have been reported throughout history. Havelock Ellis, who studied sexuality in the late nineteenth and early twentieth centuries, wrote "There is, indeed, no excretion or product of the body which has not been a source of ecstasy" to someone. It can be added that there is nothing done to or by the body that does not give someone erotic stimulation and sexual satisfaction. (Bullough & Bullough, 1977, p. 198)

Unfortunately, the early years of psychotherapy pathologized fetishes. In the late nineteenth and early twentieth centuries, professionals used harsh, judgmental terms such as "pervert" or "deviant" as official descriptions for those who engaged in fetish and other unique sexual behaviors. No wonder people with fetishes continue to distrust the psychotherapy profession!

There is an extensive list of sexual fetishes; technically, anything can be turned into a fetish item. Some of the most well-known are shoes (usually women's high heels), feet, long hair, legs, breasts, buttocks, leather clothing, smooth fabrics like silk or nylon, women's undergarments such as bras, panties and stockings, fur, urine, feces, dead bodies, certain smells, tattoos, diapers, and rubber/latex items or clothing. If you search the internet, many things that websites categorize as fetishes do not fit the technical definition. We will discuss that further in the next section, kinks.

Kinks: Everything, including the kitchen sink

Out in the world, you will encounter educated people who use the word "kink" to describe things that by technical definition belong in the category of either BDSM, fetish, or some other category. Polluting the definition of kink makes it harder to educate those who don't know what it is. Kink also bleeds across several areas of unique sexual expression, making a clear definition difficult. Kink often ends up describing multiple behaviors. I tend to define kink as sexual behaviors and preferences that are not easily categorized and different from what we consider typical sexual interest.

Let me give you a few examples. Someone who is sexually aroused by being humiliated by their partner is enjoying a kink. There is no fetish item, yet some say this activity crosses over into BDSM because of the power dynamic and emotional stimulation of the humiliation. A straight married couple who engages in "cuckolding," a situation where the wife has sex with other men, usually in front of her husband, is a type of kink. Sometimes a humiliation component is involved in this activity, so again, it can bleed into BDSM. A woman who is aroused by being in a threesome with two bisexual men is engaging in a kink. It is not specific non-genital parts of their bodies she likes, or even the power dynamic; it is a kink because the two men are sexually attracted to both her and each other *and* it is a unique situation.

People who are sexually attracted to animals or pretending to be an animal (pony, kitty or puppy play), enjoy having sex with a sleeping partner, desire to be choked (either during masturbation or by a partner), or become sexually aroused by a partner with a large age discrepancy (either much older or much younger) are really engaging in kinks. As you can see from that list, many kinks are harmless, if unusual; others stretch the boundaries of consent, which can make them problematic.

When someone tells you they enjoy kink or are kinky, it is important to explore exactly what that means for them and their own experience since the range is extremely broad.

Sexual orientation: Beyond straight, gay or bisexual

Years ago, it was believed that sexual orientation was strictly about what gender, or genders, a person was sexually attracted to. In recent years, research has demonstrated that this is a limited definition for several reasons. In the field of sexology, we are beginning to understand that the genders to which people are attracted are far more fluid than previously believed. They are not set in stone and can change over a person's lifespan.

After extensive research in the 1940s, Alfred Kinsey defined sexual orientation as the gender(s) someone was attracted to in thought, fantasy and actual sexual acts. By this definition, you were straight if you thought about, fantasized sexually, and had sex with people of the opposite gender. Someone was gay if they did the same with those of their own gender. People were somewhere on the bisexual continuum if their thoughts, sexual fantasies and acts involved both genders.

Today, some people identify as pansexual, polysexual or omnisexual. While these terms are technically the same, different people prefer different terms. They all mean that the gender of a person does not determine with whom they want to be sexual. It is the person they are attracted to, regardless of gender.

There are also people who identify as asexual, meaning they have no real sexual attraction to either gender. They may have romantic involvements, often in non-sexual relationships with deep feelings of love. You also have people who identify as "straight-ish" or "gay-ish," meaning they usually identify as one would expect, but may be attracted to and sexually involved with people who are exceptions to the rule.

If I haven't confused you enough already, there is also the phrase "straight men who have sex with men." (For you grammar fanatics, that is the correct term. Sorry.) Basically, these are men who are usually married to women, identify their sexual and romantic orientation as straight, and yet enjoy sexual encounters with other men for a variety of reasons. (Kort, 2006)

Sexual orientation is also expanding into areas that have nothing to do with gender. Research is beginning to show that adult babies/diaper fetishes, open relationships such as polyamory, and even a propensity for desiring BDSM can start at such a young age, with such strong urges and unexplained reasons, that they should be seen as sexual orientations rather than individual choices. As research continues in the area of human sexuality, much of what we now think to be true may change over time.

Different areas, common threads

BDSM, fetishes, kinks, and sexual orientation may seem like very different areas, yet they share many common threads and a great deal of overlap. Someone who is pansexual (orientation), likes to be tied up, blindfolded, and spanked (BDSM), is aroused by latex underwear (fetish), and has a propensity for threesomes (kink) has covered all the bases.

In addition to people who find themselves drawn to more than one sexual area, there are other commonalities. Each domain involves a longing for heightened levels of sensation, sexual desire, and passion as well as exploration of areas that may be considered taboo. While many people who engage in these behaviors experience the same emotional closeness as those seeking sex for relational purposes, they are also looking for the fun, recreational side of sex. People practicing BDSM often have intimate connections with their partners. Once someone with a fetish or kink can feel safe enough to share their quirk with an accepting partner, they can develop a strong emotional attachment. Since they often believe that few people will understand their desires, finding that acceptance can create deep intimacy.

Exercises

The exercises in Chapter Six and Chapter Seven are different from the rest of the book. Because there is far more information than can be covered in this book, I have given you resources to research your area(s) of interest and explore what appeals to you. The internet has allowed people desiring alternative sexual expression to connect with each other like never before. This may explain the growth in both awareness and number of people involved in alternative sexuality in recent years. However, although many great resources can be found on the internet, there are also many misleading and poorly-constructed information sources. While the list I am giving you is certainly not exhaustive, it is a good start on solid information and education.

You are welcome to research all of these; however, be aware that it will take a lot of time. I encourage you to focus your attention on the area(s) that you are considering exploring in real life. Enjoy!

BDSM
Books
There are many, many more titles. These are some I recommend:
- *BDSM Basics for Beginners: A Guide for Dominants and Submissives Starting to Explore the Lifestyle* by Michelle Fegatofi
- *When Someone You Love is Kinky* by Dossie Easton and Catherine Liszt

- *Different Loving: The World of Sexual Dominance and Submission* by Gloria & William Brame, Jon Jacobs
- *Safe, Sane, Consensual and Fun* by John Warren
- *Screw the Roses; Send Me the Thorns: The Romance and Sexual Sorcery of Sadomasochism* by Phillip Miller and Molly Devon
- *50 Shades of Kink: An Introduction to BDSM* by Tristin Taormino

Websites
- FetLife.com is a social network for the BDSM, fetish and kink communities. Like Facebook, only kinkier.
- Masters and slaves Together, International (www.MAsT.net) is a support and resource group for individuals involved or interested in the Master/slave lifestyle. The local chapters list will direct you to chapters near you.
- BDSM-101.com is an education, support and resource group with lists of books, websites, social groups, dungeons, clubs, and more.

Blogs
For those who enjoy blogs, the BDSM Blogs List (http://bdsmblogslist.kinky-blogging.com) has a comprehensive index of blogs.

Fetishes & Kinks
Because of the overlap of the term kink with both BDSM and fetishes, you will find it blended into many of the other areas.

Books
- *Fetish 101: Celebrate Your Fantasies* by Peter W. Czemich
- *Fetish Sex: An Erotic Guide for Couples* by Violet Blue & Thomas Roche

- *My Other Self: Sexual Fantasies, Fetishes and Kinks* by Angela Lewis
- *The Book of Kink: Sex Beyond the Missionary* by Eva Christina
- *Playing Well With Others: Your Field Guide to Discovering, Exploring and Navigating the Kink, Leather, and BDSM Communities* by Lee Harrington & Mollena Williams

Websites and blogs

Most fetishes have their own online communities. Search the internet for websites and blogs that cater to your particular flavor.

- Kinkacademy.com is a comprehensive library of sex-ed videos for adventurous, consenting adults. Whether you're new to kink or an experienced player, there's something for everyone to learn
- FetLife.com is a social network for the BDSM, Fetish and Kink communities. Like Facebook, only kinkier.
- Fetish-Forums.com is a social network for enthusiasts and beginners who like to explore, share and delight in the expressive art of various fetishes.
- Thefeethunter.com is a foot-fetish guide, video and dating site. It also has a top-10 list of foot fetish websites at http://thefeethunter.com/top-10-foot-fetish-websites/

Sexual Orientation

Books

- *Sexual Fluidity: Understanding Women's Love and Desire* by Lisa M. Diamond
- *Dual Attraction: Understanding Bisexuality* by Martin S. Weinberg, Colin J. Williams, & Douglas W. Pryor

Websites and blogs
- Pansexuality is Perfect http://pansexualityisperfect.tumblr.com
- Stop-homophobia.com is a site that, along with some great information, discusses pansexuality and the difference between that and bisexuality. (http://www.stop-homophobia.com/pansexuality.htm)
- Yoursexualorientation.info is a guide for people questioning their sexual orientation.
- Bisexual.org provides resources and blogs relating to bisexuality

Check in: How are you doing?

OK, that is a lot of information! Engaging in extensive research of your preferred area will take some time. Initial research will easily take weeks, yet becoming a true expert can take a lifetime. Enjoy the excitement of this initial exploration. Notice whether any Big Four negative emotions—fear, shame, guilt or embarrassment—are flaring up. If so, practice managing your emotions. Feel free to journal the mix of emotions you are feeling.

In Chapter Seven, we will continue the education and exploration with discussion of open relationships before moving on to discuss the pros and cons of unique sexual behaviors in Chapter Eight.

Chapter Seven

More Exploration

*Way beyond three's company—understanding
the wide world of open relationships*

"I'm nervous. I don't know what to expect. Will there be an orgy?
Will people be tearing my clothes off? What's going to happen?" These were some of the words, verbalized and internalized, by my (up until that point) vanilla and sexually inhibited husband as we prepared to leave for our first swinger event. To be clear, there was no orgy, no one had their clothes torn off, and he handled the event far better than he (or I) had imagined. Since the behavior of people in open relationships is relatively unknown to greater society, wild myths and misconceptions abound.

People engaging in relationship styles outside of monogamy have been successfully operating for thousands of years, if not longer. In the whole of human history, it is only in the past couple of hundred years that the belief that two people meet, fall in love, fulfill all each other's needs, and live happily ever after as soulmates has flourished. The divorce rate has been at or above 50 percent for much of the last half-century; research indicates that infidelity rates range from 40 to 70 percent, depending on how honest study participants are. Clearly there are substantial cracks in the foundation of the belief that monogamy is the best relationship style for everyone. Later in this chapter, we will explore the various sexual personality types and how for some people, monogamy is absolutely the best choice. However, since there are many personality types, we must be open to additional options.

Open relationships and non-monogamy are umbrella terms that encompass several relationship styles. These styles have many differences as well as many similarities. We will explore polyamory, where someone has more than one committed, emotionally and physically intimate relationship. We will explore swinging, or as some call it, the lifestyle, which tends to be recreational and involves less deep emotional commitment. While it was thought to be dead after the 1970s, the internet breathed new life into swinging; it is now very much alive. We will explore what some call designer relationships, which are not monogamous but do not fit the definition of polyamory or swinging, and are often unique to the people involved in them. Finally, we will discuss the concept of sexual personality types and help you understand whether you are monosexual, polysexual or an adapter.

The continuum of open relationships

If the concept of open relationships is new to you, this chapter may really stretch the way you think about relationship dynamics. Our society is so heavily weighted toward monogamy that even though alternative relationships have always been with us, they have been hidden. This can make the thought of changing one's relationship style difficult, since few people find successful examples in their families, friends, or neighbors. There is also a wide range within which these types of relationships operate. Therefore, you may know people who operate somewhere along the open-relationship continuum but who conceal this side of their lives.

There are concepts we need to discuss that will increase your understanding of various relationship choices, as well as help you decide if exploring one of them is right for you. Just like in Chapter Five when we talked about learning to grow your ability to give yourself permission, self-confidence is important. If you haven't already improved your self-confidence and you want to explore open relationships, you need to go back and work through those exercises. When taking a sexual relationship from exclusive to some version of open, self-confidence for everyone involved is very important. It can mean the difference between success and a train wreck! You need to be able to identify your wants, needs, and desires and have the confidence to communicate them to your partner, which can be a difficult conversation.

One of the terms you may hear when exploring open relationships is "compersion." This is the concept of finding pleasure in your partner's pleasure. For example, you may feel happy that your partner is enjoying a new relationship that fulfills a need you cannot provide.

That leads us to a couple of other emotions that are confusing and troublesome for people starting down this path: jealousy and envy. While these are two distinct feelings, our society has so seriously polluted the definitions that many use them incorrectly without understanding what they mean. Jealousy is the feeling that you are going to be replaced in your relationship by someone else. Envy is the wish that you could have something or engage in an activity someone else has or is doing. Here is an example: on Facebook, I see someone writing about a trip they are taking and a friend states they are jealous. Since they are not being replaced as a friend they are envious rather than jealous. Their friend is on a trip they wish they could be enjoying as well. In open relationships, it is important to understand the difference between these emotions. You may feel envious if your partner has an easier time finding another relationship than you do or if they are getting more attention from others. Again, envy is different from jealousy.

One way to handle feeling jealous when your partner finds a new partner is to ask yourself, "Am I really in jeopardy of being replaced?" Since we are usually taught that love is a finite entity when it comes to adult sexual relationships, many people mistakenly believe they are being replaced. In reality, their partner is capable of loving more than one person (it's likely that you are too). By the way, when one is excited about a new relationship, it's important to ensure that excitement does not cause you to stop giving adequate attention to your original partner. This is a common mistake I often see people make.

I like to use an analogy about the love parents have for their children to help people better understand open relationships. If you have more than one child, did you stop loving the first one when the second came along? Are you cheating on one child by paying attention to the other one? How about your third child? Just like you are capable of loving more than one child—you learn to divide your attention among them—you can love and be in love with more than one adult at a time and adapt to meet the needs of everyone involved.

As you can see, there are some definite mindset shifts that must happen to be truly successful in any open relationship. Let's look at some basic information about various types of open relationships. As in Chapter Six, the exercises at the end of this chapter will give you resources for reaching greater depth in the area(s) that have the greatest appeal to you. Before we get to the exercises, let's discuss the concept of different sexual personality types to help further educate and inform your upcoming choices.

Polyamory: Loving more than one

Polyamory (or "Poly") is the concept of having more than one emotionally and physically intimate relationship. Polyamory is very different from polygamy. Polygamy is where a man has more than one female relationship or wife. In polygamy, women are not allowed to have other male (or female) partners. There is also polyandry, where a woman has more than one male partner but the men do not have other partners. Around the world, polygamy is much more widely known and practiced than polyandry, although it does exist. In some male-dominated cultures, polyandry is practiced to keep property rights in the family; if a man dies, his brothers marry his widow. There have been cultures that practice polyandry in a way where the woman is revered, but those are less common.

Polyamory is different, and more equal, in that everyone knows about and consents to the arrangement. While not everyone in the equation chooses to have other partners, in true polyamory, everyone has the option. Relationships are out in the open and consented to by all involved, which requires a lot of open communication.

Polyamory as a term has gained prominence over the past 25 years, although the concept has been around much longer. There are numerous ways to engage in polyamory, so you may see many different configurations. A triad is where you have three people (genders can vary) who all have a sexual and romantic relationship with each other. This is similar to a couple, only with three people. The people may, or may not, all live together. A "V" is a dynamic where one person has a relationship with two others, but the other two people are not romantic or sexually involved with each other. A quad is considered two couples who have decided to have a relationship with each other. Depending on the quad, they may all be involved equally, or in a configuration unique to them.

There are many in the poly community who use the terms "primary," "secondary," or "tertiary" to identify where their different partners fall in the hierarchy of the relationship. There are others who do not want to think of their different partners being classified as more or less important to them. They reject these kinds of labels and work in a sort of non-hierarchical form.

Polyamorous relationships can take many other forms. A good resource for the various configurations can be found in Mim Chapman's book *What Does Polyamory Look Like? Polydiverse Patterns of Loving and Living in Modern Polyamorous Relationships.*

What we have discussed is more the traditional definition, but many people who identify as poly cross over into swinging and other unique, designer relationships. And even though many open relationship communities have a lot in common, they often feel that they are very different from each other and do not want to be defined by the other group's terms. If someone tells you they are in an open relationship, be sure to ask how they define themselves and do not assume they abide by the strict definition of the term. Calling a swinger poly or a poly person a swinger can get you quite a tongue lashing (and not in a fun way).

Swinging, aka "The Lifestyle"

Swinging is a form of open relationship that is usually defined as couples who engage in recreational sexual play with other couples or a single male or female. While many swingers have long-lasting friendships and sexual relationships with other singles and couples, others stick to casual sexual interactions. Those who have long-term relationships with other swingers do not look upon them as polyamory and consider their spouse their primary partner. While some people identify with the term swinger, others prefer the phrase "being in the lifestyle." There is no right or wrong, and they usually mean the same thing. As a side note, some BDSM practitioners refer to being "in the lifestyle," so be sure to clarify what it means when someone uses that term. While many people cross over and belong to both camps, others do not—and don't want to be identified as the other.

It is believed that swinging's history can be traced to an elite group of Air Force pilots and their wives in WWII. The pilots brought their wives with them when they were deployed to Europe. When they had casualties in their ranks, the other husbands began openly taking care of the needs of the widows in their group. This included their sexual needs, with their wives' knowledge and consent. This continued when they moved back to the United States and the concept of "wife swapping" was born. With the sexual openness of the 1960s and 70s, swinging flourished. It lost a lot of its luster in the 80s and 90s; but the internet renewed the practice, in large part because going online made it much easier to meet like-minded souls.

Today, if you search the internet, you will find many websites that cater to those who swing. Some sites are geographically local while others are national and international. There are also many swing clubs, resorts and cruises that cater to couples and singles who live this lifestyle.

Swingers tend to be middle to upper-middle class with families and professional careers, which can cause many to be closeted about their participation. Bisexuality among the women is almost expected, while male bisexuality has traditionally been considered taboo. Some of that has begun to change, especially within the last 10 years, and the community is beginning to be more open to various alternative sexual expressions such as BDSM, kinks, fetishes, and sexual fluidity. (Michaels & Johnson, 2015)

While men in the swinger world proudly announce that their lifestyle is all about the women and "the women rule," that has not always been my experience in the community. My husband and I have had an open marriage for about a decade and are involved in our local swinging community. While I find far more positives than negatives, my humble opinion as a strong feminist is that conventional attitudes about gender roles prevail in the lifestyle, and women tend to focus on pleasing men more than the reverse. There are certainly exceptions, and I hope to see more in time.

Historically, the belief was that the male partner initiated the idea of swinging for the couple while it was the female who kept them there. For many women, swinging offers the freedom to enjoy and explore their sexuality in a way traditional marriage and society never encouraged. Currently, that belief is being challenged. A survey conducted by the website Openminded.com concluded that in opposite-gendered couples, approximately two-thirds of those who initiated the idea of opening up their relationship were women, not men. I can only hope that this is proof that women are starting to take more control of their own sexual pleasure and destiny.

People might experiment with both swinging and polyamory, but feel that they don't quite fit in either community. This is where designer relationships come into play.

Designer relationships: Unique configurations of open

I wish I could say I created the term "designer relationship," but I cannot. I first heard it a few years back at a sex therapy training. I have always thought it was a perfect term, as I have encountered multiple people who do not quite fit into the traditional definitions of other open relationship styles, yet are successfully navigating configurations that work for those involved.

The term is credited to Kenneth Haslam, MD, founder of the Kinsey Institute's Polyamory Archive. The definition means that you and your partner or partners are the designers of your unique relationship. This relationship is designed to work for those involved and may need to be redesigned as time goes on. Designer relationship is an inclusive term that encompasses people who bond emotionally but not sexually; those who choose to be sexually exclusive; those who choose to be sexually nonexclusive; those with occasional lovers or friends with benefits; multiple partner configurations with long-term bonds; and partnerships in which certain kinky activities take place outside the primary relationship. It can include being single by choice, single and either poly or swinging, asexual, nonsexual, monogamous by choice (rather than expectation), semi-consensual non-monogamy, and friends with benefits, to name a few. (Michaels & Johnson, 2015)

I have seen designer relationships where couples have discussed and understood that the partner who needs more sexual variety has the option to see others occasionally. This happens even if the other partner never uses the same option or wants to know the details of the extra-relationship encounters. Usually there is an understanding that the one who engages in other sexual relationships will use safer sex protections and get tested from time to time to limit exposure and transmission of sexually-transmitted infections to their primary partner.

Designer relationships can also include people who mostly fit into the poly world but desire some recreational sexual activities, and swingers who engage in some level of deeper commitment or polyamory. It can also work for partners where one tends to prefer sex in a committed relationship while their primary partner enjoys recreational sexual encounters outside of the primary relationship. As you can imagine, there are as many ways of designing an open relationship as there are people having relationships.

Sexual personality types

A few voices in the field of sexology are beginning to define the concept of sexual personality types. After exposure to these new thoughts, along with groundbreaking research I have read and my academic, clinical and personal exposure, I am now presenting the concept of sexual personality types to a larger audience. Although more extensive research is needed, I believe there is enough evidence currently to begin discussing this concept.

This theory accepts that just like other personality types, there are unique sexual personality types that people either develop or are born with. These fall into three categories: monosexual, polysexual, or adapter. Let's explore them a bit deeper.

Someone who is monosexual is best suited to exclusive sexual and romantic relationships such as traditional monogamy. As long as they are paired with another monosexual individual, their relationship works well, at least from the sexual aspect. Monosexuals paired with adapters can also work well, but if they are paired with a polysexual individual, there is trouble on the sexual front.

A person is polysexual when they're most comfortable in some form of open relationship. As we just explored, there are many models for what an open relationship can look like. Some people realize they are polysexual at a young age and engage in open relationships from the beginning. Most polysexual people attempt to meet the social expectations of monogamy. Once paired with a monosexual person, they find themselves straying from (or feeling confined by) the expected boundaries. When allowed to engage in some form of consensual non-monogamy, they usually flourish, since this fits their personality type.

An exception to this is someone who has cheated on their partner in a monogamous relationship and does it again in an open relationship. It is possible to cheat in an open relationship; I have seen it happen. Sometimes a person's choice to seek other sexual partners is different from being polysexual. Some people enjoy the thrill and taboo of sneaking around and hiding something from their partner. They think having an open relationship will solve the problem, but it doesn't. They find they cannot help themselves because they enjoy doing things they are not supposed to do. That is a different animal than the polysexual type who does well with consensual open relationships.

Finally, we have the adapters. In my professional experience, most people are either monosexual or polysexual, but there are a few people who can happily exist in either a monogamous or open relationship. I call these people adapters because they can go from an exclusive relationship to an open relationship, then back to an exclusive relationship. Adapters do not seem to miss the unique dynamics of the other. Most monosexual or polysexual types cannot make this type of change without some resentment or unhappiness.

Here is an example. I worked with a couple where one person was monosexual and one was polysexual. They had started their relationship as monogamous; soon afterwards, he initiated the idea of an open relationship. For a few years it appeared to be going well. There were signs along the way that she was not completely onboard—she usually had to consume a lot of alcohol to engage with other couples—and eventually the truth came out. She wanted to return to their original monogamous arrangement. He was shocked and not happy about going back to monogamy.

However, due to his love for her and dedication to their marriage, he chose to give up the open side of the relationship. There was a cost for this decision as he was sometimes resentful and definitely less than happy. At times, this would bleed into their relationship and make them both unhappy. This example shows how each was clearly a unique sexual personality type. And despite exposure to both options, neither was the elusive adapter.

Since this is a relatively new theory in the field of sexology, there is no scientifically vetted assessment test for you to take to find out which type you fall into. Maybe someday we will have one. For the time being, here are some questions and thoughts for you to ponder to help give you more information in your decision-making about your sexual personality type.

1. Look back over the various sexual and romantic relationships you have experienced in your life. If they have always been exclusive, was that by design or assumed expectation?

2. Were there any incidents of infidelity, whether they were discovered or kept secret? Would you have behaved differently if you could have experienced other relationships with your partner's knowledge and consent? How would you have felt about your partner having other sexual partners?

3. If you did engage in any open situations with your partner and another couple or single man or woman; were you sober or did you have to be drunk or high in order to do it?

4. If you have been in both exclusive and open relationships, were you happy in both? Would the relationship style of your next relationship matter to you? Would either style be comfortable to you or would you prefer one over the other?

Notice your answers to these questions. While not definitive, it can give you an idea if you may be monosexual, polysexual, or an adapter.

The various types of open relationships: Similarities and distinct differences

We have covered a lot of information in this chapter and to be honest, this is just an overview. As you will see from the resources listed in the exercises, there is a great deal more to learn about open relationship styles. There are also a lot of nuances and mindset shifts that must take place in order to successfully navigate any of these relationship dynamics.

At their core, open relationships are similar in that they have the informed consent and knowledge of those involved in them. Even people who choose not to have other sexual partners are aware of and consent to their primary partner having other types of sexual and romantic partners.

The differences come when we look at things like how casual and recreational relationships are versus the levels of emotional bonding and connection. Some in the swinging world never have sex with the same additional partners twice. Some in the polyamory world have two or more partners who are committed to each other for decades or even a lifetime.

Some people understand the sexual personality type early on in their relationship history and choose to be exclusive or open by choice, rather than fall into monogamy by default. Most people learn about their true sexual personality type after painful experiences of exploration, infidelity, and broken promises that ended relationships—or at least damaged them.

Look back over your own relationship history as well as the history of your close friends and confidants. What patterns do you see? Have you been longing for something other than what society and those around you thought was the right choice? Or have your relationship dynamics felt like a perfect fit?

Exercises

The exercises for this chapter are opportunities to further your knowledge in the area of open relationships.

Following are a list of books, websites and blogs to help you learn more about what we have discussed. Like Chapter Six, this is not an exhaustive list; it is meant to get you started and give you a solid level of education and information. This will help with your decision-making later on.

Swinging/The Lifestyle
Books

- *Swinging Lifestyle Superbook: Couples Swap Spouses* by Tony Kelbrat
- *Swinging for beginners: An Introduction to the Lifestyle* by Kaye Bellemeade
- *Swinging 101: A Couple's Lifestyle Primer* by Andre Keith
- *Swingers' Lifestyle: The Questions You are Afraid to Ask* by Jacki Melfi

Websites, information and dating

- Swingers.org offers a variety of articles about the lifestyle and is an important source of information.
- Kasidie.com: this site and the sites below it are a good way to find other swingers, clubs and events as well as helpful blogs and discussion boards.
- Swinglifestyle.com: (aka SLS.com)
- Swingers Date Club: (aka SDC.com)

Resorts, clubs and travel

- Hedonism Resort, www.hedonism.com. A resort in Jamaica that caters to nudists and swingers.
- Desire Resort and Spa www.desire-resort.com. A resort south of Cancun, Mexico in the Rivera Maya that caters to nudists and swingers.

Swing clubs

There are many small swing clubs across the country. Check your local area for those close to you. Here is a small list of some of the most noteworthy.

- The Scarlet Ranch, Denver, CO
- New Horizons Adult Social Club, Seattle, WA
- Sea Mountain Nude Resort and Spa, Desert Hot Springs, CA
- Trapeze, Atlanta, GA and Ft. Lauderdale, FL
- Miami Velvet, Miami, FL
- Colette, New Orleans, LA

Travel agencies

- Theswingercruise.com is an agency that deals with cruises, resorts and other areas of lifestyle vacations. It is my personal favorite. If you call, tell Lynn I said "hello." She and her staff are amazing!
- Toplesstravel.com is affiliated with SLS.com. It is a very good service and the staff are knowledgeable.
- Luxury Lifestyle Vacations (LLV), www.luxury-lifestyle-vacations.com is a site catering to upper-middle class and above clientele.

Polyamory
Books

- *The Ethical Slut: A Practical Guide to Polyamory, Open Relationships and Other Adventures* by Dossie Easton and Janet Hardy. This is a must-read for anyone starting down the open relationship path.
- *Opening Up: A Guide to Creating and Sustaining Open Relationships* by Tristan Taormino

- *More Than Two: Polyamory Resources and Guidelines* by Eve Rickert
- *Polyamory: The New Love Without Limits: Secrets of Sustainable Intimate Relationships* by Deborah Anapol

Websites and blogs

- Lovingmore.com is an educational and advocacy resource for polyamory and open relationships.
- Morethantwo.com is a good site for those exploring and wanting more information.
- Polyamorysociety.org is a non-profit organization that promotes and supports those in open relationships.
- Polyinthemedia.blogspot.com tracks the coverage of polyamory in the media.
- Meetup.com helps users find local groups for meeting and discussing the polyamory lifestyle.

Designer relationships

Books

- *Designer Relationships: A Guide to Happy Monogamy, Positive Polyamory, and Optimistic Open Relationships* by Mark A. Michaels and Patricia Johnson
- *Mating in Captivity: Unlocking Erotic Intelligence* by Esther Perel
- *The New Monogamy and Getting the Sex You Want* by Tammy Nelson
- *The Sex and Love Handbook: Polyamory! Bisexuality! Swingers! Spirituality! (& even) Monogamy! A Practical, Optimistic Relationship Guide* by Kris & Rozz Heinlein

Thinking about sexuality differently

Books

- *Sex Outside the Lines: Authentic Sexuality in a Sexually Dysfunctional Culture by Chris Donaghue*
- *Modern Sexuality: The Truth About Sex and Relationships* by Michael Aaron
- *Sex at Dawn: How We Mate, Why We Stray, and What it Means for Modern Relationships* by Christopher Ryan & Cacilda Jetha

Check in: How are you doing?

Wow! The past two chapters have covered a lot of vital information. I hope you are not overwhelmed. It is a huge amount to take in and learn. In Chapter Eight we will examine the pros and cons of open relationships, BDSM, fetishes, kinks, and the newest view of sexual orientation. We will also explore the process of adapting your sex and relationship mindset to help give you a foundation for success if you decide to explore new relationship dynamics.

Learning the Pros and Cons

How to enjoy yourself and avoid the landmines

I know many people in both my professional practice and personal
life who conduct their sexual relationships differently than much
of society. These people have successfully created new ways to enjoy
their sexuality. I've witnessed the joy that can come from these suc-
cesses. I've also seen the pain that results from mistakes, which are
easy to make as you change the way you live your life. Most of us
grow up with a monogamy mindset; when we change our behavior,
our mindset needs to change as well. If those do not evolve, we continue to use our monosexual mindset, which conflicts with our new
lifestyle.

In this chapter, I will serve as a guide to help you navigate the
process of adapting your mindset along with your behaviors. I will
point out some of the landmines I have often seen people step on.

I have always believed that it is easier to learn from other people's mistakes than to have to repeat them myself. Here is an opportunity for you to learn from those mistakes and explore the fun things to look forward to while embarking on your new journey.

Open relationships: Pros and cons

As we learned in Chapter Seven, open relationships cover a wide range of lifestyles; the pros and cons of their various configurations can vary. Overall, many of the advantages and disadvantages are similar, but some are unique to swinging, polyamory, or designer relationships.

Pros

One of the greatest advantages people find in open relationships is a sense of variety. This variety can be from the obvious source—having sex with other people—as well as fulfilling non-sexual needs a primary partner is unable to fulfill. Many are surprised to find that sexual variety can ignite new excitement in their primary relationship. Sex with the same person day after day and year after year can become stale even for inventive partners.

Adding variety, if only occasionally, can stoke the fires of passion between people even if they were nearly burned out. As those who engage in sex with others discover, different partners can be surprising. Different doesn't mean they no longer enjoy their original partner, and different doesn't mean better. But varied ways of flirting, touching, kissing, or performing sexual acts can open up a world of excitement and possibilities. Sometimes you learn new things to bring home and share with your primary partner!

There is also a benefit to open relationships when the people in the original relationship have very different levels of libido. The higher-libido partner can find other high-libido partners, which takes pressure off the lower-libido partner. Sometimes the lower-libido partner's desire increases once they feel that they can wait until they desire sex. Usually, this increase is still not as high as their primary partner, so having other outlets works well for both as long as they continue to meet the main needs of the relationship.

Another advantage of variety is being free to engage in sexual activities that your partner doesn't enjoy, want to do, or is simply unable to do. By unable, I mean things like changing their gender, if you enjoy being with another gender, or being two different people if you enjoy threesomes. If there are kinks, fetishes, or BDSM activities you desire but your partner does not, this gives you an opportunity to enjoy what you like without your partner feeling obligated to take one for the team.

Another unexpected advantage many find is a much deeper sense of intimacy with their primary partner once they open the relationship. While this might seem counterintuitive, being able to have more honest conversations about sexual wants and receiving acceptance for them can bring people closer. In all sexual relationships, the ideal expectation is "Here is a person with whom I can truly be myself and be vulnerable," which should lead to better intimacy. Yet based on what I have seen from most monogamous couples, this expectation is rarely met because they fear rejection if they are truly honest about their needs and desires.

No matter how in love or compatible one may feel with a partner, one person can rarely fulfill all of another's wants, needs and desires. Those who engage in polyamorous relationships find this to be an advantage. Each partner is appreciated for their unique contributions and it can lessen resentment when a partner doesn't fulfill a need that another partner does.

Cons

Many fear that opening their relationship will destroy it. As I like to say, "Open relationships will not destroy a solid relationship and will not save one with a cracked foundation." A common problem I see when a couple opens up their marriage is they do it because they want someone, anyone, other than their original partner. If your relationship is on the verge of divorce, opening the relationship is unlikely to save it. I say "unlikely" because I have seen marriages on the verge of divorce saved when they are opened up. I tend to see this as the exception; however, it does happen.

One huge disadvantage of open relationships (as with all alternative sexuality lifestyle choices) is that most people around you will not understand. People are quick to judge what they don't understand, and many in your social circle may judge you harshly (or at least be confused) about what makes this so important to you. While it shouldn't matter what other people think, the fact is that it does matter for many people. This causes people to hide their sexual lifestyle choices out of fear of judgment and rejection. I have seen people lose friends, family members and intimate relationships when they finally come out as their authentic selves. Depending on the people around you, this might be the price you must pay.

This disapproval and judgement of your lifestyle can lead to discrimination in employment, being shunned by the neighbors and, especially for polyamorous people, problems in divorce and child custody cases with a previous monogamous partner. Many people in poly relationships as well as those who swing grapple with how to talk to, or whether to tell, their children. For those who are poly, it can be difficult to hide another committed partner, especially if everyone wants to live together. Many people learn to manage it, and some of the resources from Chapter Seven will give you ways to deal with this complicated issue.

Many swingers hide their sexual relationships from their children and, depending on the ages of the children, this choice is certainly acceptable. After all, how many monogamous couples give their young children details of their sexual behaviors? Problems can arise as children become teens, grow more computer-savvy, and find their parents' internet history. What is there to say about a browser history that includes"theswingercruise.com?" That can be tough to explain.

Another common issue people face is that open relationships force them to tackle their own insecurities. Fear of not being good enough, attractive enough, sexually skilled enough—the list goes on and on—can cripple people emotionally. Before recognizing the depth of one's insecurity or how to get control of it, emotional flare-ups with a partner can heighten fears about whether the couple is on the right path. In time, this can be turned into an advantage if you are able to explore a painful emotional process. Working through irrational emotional responses can give you better clarity regarding everything you were taught at a young age. If you are not able to recognize and tweak these ingrained beliefs, they can destroy or seriously damage your relationship.

Finally, what many consider a disadvantage is the added risk of unintended pregnancy or sexually-transmitted infections. When you have more than one sexual partner, your STI risk certainly increases. However, there are ways to limit your exposure with consistent use of either male or female condoms and contraception to prevent pregnancy from anyone other than your primary partner.

Some studies have shown that for an unknown reason, there is a lower incident of sexually transmitted infections within the organized swinger community. It may be because many in this community use protection more consistently than the general population. Eventually, it comes down to the level of risk one is willing to take.

Consider the other levels of risk in your life. If you drive without wearing a seatbelt, fly down an eight-lane freeway 10 or 20 mph over the speed limit, smoke, overindulge in alcohol or recreational drugs, eat an unhealthy diet and have a sedentary life, STIs are the least of your concern. I don't mean to be flippant, but so often people allow their anxiety and fears about STIs to grow out of proportion to the actual risk. Use protection, but do not overreact to the real risk.

BDSM: Pros and cons
Pros
In Chapter Six, we saw the tip of the iceberg that is BDSM. If this is an area where you did further research, you now know much more and are probably already aware of its basic pros and cons.

Similar to open relationships, one of the advantages of BDSM is that it allows people to explore and express both sexual and personality desires which tend to be frowned upon in general society. The person who enjoys inflicting pain on a person who enjoys submitting to pain now feels at home and surrounded by like-minded souls. For various reasons, many people find pain to be a level of physical stimulation that they crave and desire. When they find others who understand, accept, and can help them explore these desires, it can create a sense of normalcy. When you have felt the need to hide your desires, even from those closest to you, finding that level of acceptance can be liberating.

Those who become an active part of their local BDSM community will find other accepting people. They will also meet educated people who have learned proper technique for unique behaviors and situations, and who are often more than willing to share their vast knowledge. Local clubs and dungeons often offer classes and workshops on proper techniques as well as how to handle certain emotional and psychological aspects that can occur during the intensity of the emotional and physical sensations which both the dominant side and submissive side often experience.

Cons

One of the cons is that there can be a lack of approval or judgment from others. This depends on several factors, including where you live. If you live in a small or conservative community, the issue of disapproval, discrimination, and judgment can be very real. There are even some states where it is illegal to strike a consenting partner, making consensual BDSM illegal. It can also depend on other people's experiences in life. If someone has experienced real abuse or domestic violence, they may mistake BDSM for the same. With some education, you may be able to help them see the very distinct differences, yet for others this will trigger too many painful memories for them to understand.

BDSM has been used against people when they get involved in divorce and child custody cases, even if the other partner was a consenting participant at the time. How often have you heard of someone stating after the fact that they were coerced or pressured into doing something when in reality, they enthusiastically consented? While people can be coerced into participating in BDSM, more often than not in these particular cases it is a tactic to win sympathy from an under-educated judge.

Many who engage in consensual BDSM are reluctant to talk to their doctor about marks on their bodies from spanking, flogging, caning, or other practices out of fear they will be seen as victims of abuse and reported to social services or law enforcement. More healthcare professionals and emergency personnel are being educated about the differences between real abuse and consensual BDSM. Again, it depends on where you live. If you live in a smaller community and/or your medical provider is uneducated about consensual

BDSM, a good resource to give them is *Health Care Without Shame: A Handbook for the Sexually Diverse and Their Caregivers* by Dr. Charles Moser.

Fetishes and Kinks: Pros and cons
Pros

Even though fetishes and kinks are technically different, they share enough similarities in their pros and cons to combine them in this discussion. Fetishes tend to develop during childhood and usually begin to show up by puberty. While some people with kinks mention a preference for unique behaviors once they become sexually active, many more discover their kinks after hearing about it or having it introduced to them by a sexual partner.

Once people embrace the unique sexual behaviors of fetishes and kinks, they can achieve levels of comfort and personal acceptance they have never felt before. Most feel intense shame and embarrassment related to their sexual interests and so self-acceptance can be difficult. But once achieved, freedom from negative emotions is liberating. Many people who have fetishes and kinks have more than one, so giving oneself permission to accept one fetish or kink can open up exploration of others.

In addition, once someone has self-acceptance, it is much easier to find partners who enjoy, or are willing try, the same sexual flavors. And since a new, accepting partner may have other kinks, this can expand one's sexual horizons. This can continue to make sex fun, exciting, and even more mentally and physically stimulating.

Cons

Attaining true self-acceptance can be difficult. I have worked with people for whom this process took years and is something they continually need to manage. Due to the intensity of negative emotions for those with fetishes and kinks, it is easy for them to doubt that anyone will ever accept them and their desired sexual behaviors. This causes people to hide their behaviors, only bringing them out with sex workers (which can become expensive) or surprising their partners without explaining their fetish or kink. An uneducated partner rarely handles this situation well when it is sprung upon them, which further emotionally damages the person with the fetish/kink and convinces them that they're the one with the problem.

At the end of the day, it is fear of rejection that causes most people with fetishes and kinks to hide their behaviors, which reinforces their negative beliefs about themselves. Once ingrained, this can be challenging to correct. As a therapist, it can be difficult to convince someone things can be different when experience has told them otherwise.

To avoid this, I talk with people about how to inform and educate a new or long-term partner to help avoid severe negative experiences that then imprint the belief that they are bad, flawed, or some sort of freak. While not always successful, I have found educating their partner, in a neutral place and at a non-sexual time, will go a long way towards a better outcome. It can be helpful to share with your partner what these fetishes or kinks give you as far as sexual excitement and pleasure. This can be difficult, as many with these types of alternative expression having difficulty understanding their own desires. Even if you struggle to understand your kink or fetish yourself, letting your partner know that s/he is still important to you, and that you want to explore this unique quirk together, can go a long way towards a better understanding.

New view of sexual orientation: Pros and cons
Pros

The relatively recent expanded view of sexual orientation has many advantages for those who have felt different or marginalized most of their lives. When someone has a sexual desire at odds with how they were raised and what they were taught was "normal," learning that their feelings are due to their orientation, rather than a choice, can be refreshing. Those who are bisexual, pansexual, asexual, or have always felt a propensity towards polyamory, BDSM, or kink can feel vindicated and gain a sense that they belong because of advances in our thinking about orientation.

There are also huge advantages that acceptance brings in giving people permission to discover their true selves. For many, this exploration can bring fun and excitement back to sex when it appeared to be over years ago. Acceptance of orientation, as with all unique sexual expressions, means that we are able to meet others who think like we do and learn far more about what we can mean and become.

Cons

Embracing a new understanding of your orientation may result in the feeling that you are constantly educating everyone around you. Until Miley Cyrus publicly came out as pansexual, most people had never heard the term and in many smaller, more conservative communities, many still have not heard it. If you are poly, many will consider this a choice and the need to educate your neighbors, friends, family, co-workers, children's teachers, and so on can seem daunting.

If you are in a relationship with someone and have hidden this part of yourself for many years, coming out to them can also be difficult. The excitement of discovering your true orientation can come to a crashing halt when you realize you have to tell your long-term partner and face their reaction. Your newly-expressed orientation might seem like liberal, academic rubbish to your partner, and they may want you to go back to hiding your true self from the world. There can be great pressure from family and friends to behave how they thought you always were and should be. It can take strength to rise up and be who you really are despite the views of others. We will cover this further in the final chapters, so don't feel you have to conquer this quite yet.

Your new sexual mindset: Thinking about sex and relationships differently

As you begin to behave differently in sex and relationships, you will bump up against your old sexual mindset. While your thoughts and beliefs will evolve during the process of accepting and embracing your new sexual self, there will be some that are so deeply ingrained you didn't even realize they were there. At some point, one of those will hit you right between the eyes and you will be forced to deal with it.

Your beliefs about acceptable gender roles will most likely come into play. Even if you were raised with more liberal gender roles or have pushed yourself to evolve your beliefs, these can still come into play. When people think of BDSM, most envision a man in the dominant role with a female in the submissive role. I have been told by a very credible source (one of my BDSM clients) that for every male dominant, there are two female submissives in the BDSM community. Yet for every female dominant, there are four or five male submissives. Not quite the stereotype!

The monosexual beliefs that are deeply instilled by an overwhelmingly monogamous culture will be ones you will certainly encounter if you choose to have any form of open relationship. The whole concept of soulmates or finding "the one" is very strong, so watching your partner have open feelings of love, or even lust, for another person can feel very threatening.

I have often heard how threatening it can feel for people to see and hear their partner have sex with someone else. Their partner may move differently, make new noises, or have stronger orgasms than they have ever had with them! It is OK for this to feel weird or uncomfortable. However, it does not mean your primary partner no longer loves and adores you, or is secretly planning to leave you for another. Different people invoke varied levels and intensity of sexual chemistry.

Veronica and her husband bumped into this when she started seeing a mutual friend. She and this person had intense sexual chemistry, were good friends, and that was *all*. Even if they had wanted to be more, they would have been lousy relationship partners. Her husband misinterpreted the intense sexual chemistry to mean deep love and feared their marriage was going to end. He began acting odd and making statements that were out of character for him. Once Veronica realized what he feared, she was able to assure him that she had no plans to leave him for this man or any other that she knew of. Once they cleared this up, life went back to normal.

People in polyamorous relationships must rethink relationship dynamics, especially when they decide to live together. You must decide how to deal with family holidays, neighbors, children's friends and teachers, and the day-to-day of who sleeps with whom and how often. The process of learning to live with a person is stressful enough when it is only two people; add one or two more, and the stress can increase during this adjustment period.

It is not possible to give you all the ways to change your sex and relationship mindset. Hopefully, this has given you some idea of what you may encounter and how to react. Realize that unexpected beliefs will come up. It can be a bit easier to manage when you understand that you will step on some landmines no matter how well you plan. When that happens, take a deep breath, realize what it is, and find a way to talk about it. Calmly discussing it in the open is always better than holding it in or yelling and blaming others for your emotions.

Exercises

After the huge amount of information in the previous three chapters, it is time for some additional journaling. By now, I am guessing you have narrowed the area(s) you have interest in exploring or expressing. Write down your thoughts about what you envision will be some positive aspects for you. Also, be sure to give some thought to possible pitfalls or challenges that you recognize. Try not to allow the possible pitfalls and challenges to scare you off. For now, just recognize them.

Check in: How are you doing?

Are you feeling more excited and strong after learning about embracing your new sexual self, or are your negative emotions creeping back in? Hopefully you have far more excitement and happy thoughts about moving forward. The next couple of chapters will give you a chance to begin to test the waters (if you haven't already) as well as face any difficult decisions you may have to make as a result of embracing your sexual and relationship choices.

Chapter Nine

Testing the Waters

Do you dip your toes in or dive into the deep end?

"**D**r. Rhoda, you are not going to believe what happened. I am so excited I couldn't wait to see you so I could tell you all about it!" I have to admit that I love watching people test the waters after finally giving themselves permission to explore. Their level of excitement can be difficult to describe, but I love to listen as they tell me the details of their new adventures. Since they often cannot discuss this with many people in their lives, the few who are privy to their new lives get all the fun details. We also get the responsibility of responding to wide-eyed pleas for help about how to improve mistakes or meet challenges. This period of exploration is filled with fun and excitement as well as difficulties. It will test people far more than they realize and help them understand if this is really the path they want to go down.

Testing the waters of a new sexual or relationship style can be both an exciting and terrifying time. There can be great excitement because you are finally able to do the things you have only imagined. This can create an intoxicating and overwhelming bundle of emotions. Often people feel like a kid locked in a candy store, wanting to try a little of everything.

Sometimes this level of overwhelming excitement can cause people to make decisions they wouldn't make when they are thinking more clearly. It can cause some of the disadvantages we discussed in the last chapter, such as failing to give their primary partner enough attention during this thrilling new time of being allowed to have new partners.

Some people have tested the waters numerous times in the past and understand that they want these changes, but fear of being their true selves continues to stop them. Practicing the techniques for managing negative emotions we discussed in Chapter Two and the confidence-building steps in Chapter Five can help you succeed this time around.

For those who felt they wanted *something* different, yet allowed their fear to stop them from even exploring the options, this is your time. We have worked on managing your negative emotions as well as building your confidence and permission to explore. You have a great deal of information to explore about common alternative sexual and relationship styles. Now is the time for both those who know what they want and those who suspect what they want to get out there.

In this chapter, I will share more details from the people whose stories we have been following along the way and give you more information about their journeys. We will examine what they learned, as well as what you can learn from their experiences, both positive and negative. At the end of the chapter, I will give you exercises (along with a little push) to get out and begin to really explore.

If you are currently in a committed relationship and have not told your partner about your desires and exploration, I have some thoughts. While I am neither condemning nor condoning sexual encounters outside your committed relationship without your partner's knowledge, I am also a realist. Sometimes you need to do your own exploration to know whether this is the best path for you. This exploration helps you understand how to approach your partner.

For some, sex outside of their primary relationship is very black-and-white; they do not want to cheat on their partner. I certainly understand and respect that belief. If you feel like you cannot dip your toes in too far without first disclosing to your partner, please read Chapter 10 before engaging in a deeper level of exploration. This will help guide decision-making such as whether to explore without your partner's expressed knowledge or postpone exploring until you make tough choices about the long-term feasibility of your current relationship.

David: A Dominant meets his submissive

As you may remember, David's BDSM desires had been bubbling over into his life and he was afraid to tell his traditional vanilla wife about his long-hidden desires. Once he finally confided in his wife, he learned that his suspicions were true—this was not something she wanted to explore with him. David needed an additional partner with whom to engage in BDSM behaviors. Since they didn't want to divorce, they decided to open their relationship to some form of designer relationship or polyamory. Transitioning from a traditional, monogamous relationship to an open one was no easy task. It involved many therapy sessions, both as a couple and individually. We did a great deal of work to help them sort through the emotions as well as the mindset shifts that had to happen for them to be successful.

Now David's BDSM desires were out in the open and accepted as a part of himself. Knowing the genie could not be put back in the bottle, his wife had two options. We discussed them many times during this process. She could file for divorce and search for a new partner who was a monosexual personality like her, or she could wrap her head around the new relationship dynamics. While she struggled with the thought of her husband having another sexual partner, her desire to maintain her marriage was stronger than anything else. I often wondered, to myself, if they would make it through this process. However, the choice to continue their marriage, even though it was now different, was more important to both than starting over.

Once they made it over this hurdle, David could start exploring. He quickly found a woman who shared many of his feelings about BDSM. She was also a sexual submissive.

What David and his wife learned was that their marriage and commitment to each other was stronger than either of them realized. Even though his wife did not want to redefine their sexual and relationship dynamics, when given the option, she chose to stay and learn how to adapt rather than leave the marriage. After working with them so intensely, I learned that one never knows what choices people will make until they're faced with them. Many others would have chosen to get divorced. However, these two found that renegotiating their relationship, while difficult, was the best option.

Josh: A fetish out of hiding

Josh and his wife were at an impasse. Despite both individual and couples' counseling, they were unable to agree on a middle ground that worked for each of them. As you may remember, once she learned Josh found other women's feet and shoes sexually attractive, she would no longer let him play with her feet in a sexual manner as they had done earlier in their relationship. She was upset when she found him looking at shoe catalogs; this fed her insecurity about comparing her feet to other women's. Rather than work through her insecurities, it was easier for her to shut down this aspect of their sex life. And since this was an important part of Josh's sexuality that was not going to change, it left him with few options.

Even though Josh was becoming more and more unhappy in the marriage, he did not want to get divorced. because it might have negative ramifications for their children. The effects of divorce on children can be difficult to gauge. Different situations and ages of the children can affect their reactions.

Research tends to show that the biggest factor effecting children during divorce is how the adults involved handle the situation. If parents allow their pain and anger over the divorce to bleed into their interactions with their children, talk badly about the other parent, or have an "I will destroy everything" attitude, of course they'll be negatively affected. If divorcing parents have a "We are the adults and need to behave accordingly" attitude and can work together to co-parent despite their differences, the children do much better.

In therapy, we discussed how Josh's fetish was not something that would go away. We talked about the increasing chasm between him and his wife and considered how to minimize the damage of a divorce on their children. Even though this was not his first choice, he decided to see what a trial separation would bring.

I often tell people that when two sides cannot find resolution, a separation can bring about answers. It does not necessarily lead to divorce and sometimes may save a marriage. While it may not give both sides the answers they want, it *will* provide answers. This can be very frightening to people, since they do not know whether it will save or end the marriage.

For Josh, the answer that came in time was that in his case, divorce was the best option. This meant that as he went forward, he had to be upfront about the importance of his fetish once he started the process of finding a new sexual and romantic relationship.

Josh learned that despite his strong desire to keep his marriage and family intact, he had to be true to himself. Sexual fetishes do not go away. The best course of action is acceptance; not only self-acceptance, but acceptance by the partner. This requires a willingness to negotiate ways to have the needs of the fetish met along with the other partner's sexual needs. Both sides need to give. However, middle ground is not something that people live in for only a short time. For it to work effectively, middle ground must be a place where each person has enough comfort to remain as the relationship continues.

Veronica: Opening up a marriage

Veronica felt incredible guilt for "cheating" on her husband. Her father had cheated on her mother many times and it was something she had promised herself she would never do. However, the complete lack of sex in her otherwise wonderful marriage was more than she could bear. I often tell people that when it comes to cheating, everyone has their breaking point. Some have yet to find that breaking point, but I believe nearly everyone has one.

The man with whom she had an affair was in a similar situation. Evan had been married for many years and had not had sex with his wife since their son was born. Evan's son was 11, and while unhappy about the arrangement, he didn't want to push for sex his wife didn't want and he didn't want to leave his marriage.

Since Veronica also didn't want to leave her marriage, this appeared, at first, to be a perfect situation. They both had equally adventurous sexual spirits and began to try things that both had only imagined. One day, Evan suggested they try swapping sexually with another couple. They both agreed to experiment with the promise that if one or the other didn't like it, they could return to being involved sexually with just each other. To their happy surprise, both enjoyed it very much and decided to continue sharing their sex life with other couples from time to time.

This new level of sexual freedom led Veronica to tell her husband about the affair and ask for a separation so both of them could decide what they wanted. While her husband initially fought her on the separation and promised he would change, she had heard this too many times before and knew if she stayed nothing would change. Divorce was the last thing she wanted. She loved her husband more deeply than she had in a relationship with any other man who loved and adored her to the depth that he did.

They were separated for over a year. During this time, they frequently attempted to talk about what they wanted and needed to make the marriage work better for both of them. Veronica's husband's answer was usually "I don't know." She told him about her involvement in swinging and her enjoyment of her newfound sexual freedom. She didn't think swinging was something he would ever consider sharing with her.

After more than a year, he finally said the words she wanted and needed to hear. He wanted to put their marriage back together and find a middle ground where they both could comfortably exist. Much to their surprise, he was far more comfortable with swinging than either imagined and this new level of openness increased his sexual desire.

While Veronica felt great guilt, her affair taught her many things about herself, her sexual personality, and her best relationship style. Even though she had always engaged in monogamous relationships, she came to learn that it was out of expectation rather than choice. As she looked back on past relationships, this newfound knowledge helped her understand the many times she'd felt confined by expectations of monogamy. Previously, she had felt guilty about wanting just sex from someone new while keeping her primary relationship.

Veronica also had kinks that had been a part of her sexuality since her late teens. Despite knowing she had these desires for many years, she had never experienced them. She never gave herself permission to explore what these feelings meant earlier in her life. Most men she had mentioned them to didn't understand her unique desires, so it was easy for her to continue to hide them and judge her desires and herself. Now, with the support of her primary relationship firmly in hand and permission to explore, she was enjoying her sexuality like never before.

Veronica's husband had always been in monogamous relationships without considering anything different. He was happy they had put their marriage back together, excited to explore, and unsure where this new journey together would lead. He was learning a lot of new things and having experiences that, up until then, he had only imagined.

Evan: A marriage must end

You may be wondering what happened to Evan, the man with whom Veronica had her affair. Like her, he also separated from his wife of 20 years. They went to a marriage counselor to see if they could find middle ground. His wife believed there was nothing wrong with her for no longer wanting sex after their child had been born; she was unwilling to explore options where they both could live equally. She no longer desired sex and thought Evan shouldn't, either. Although they had not had sex for more than a decade, she was extremely upset that he had sought it elsewhere.

Before his affair with Veronica, Evan had satisfied his sexual needs with short-term sexual encounters. After the affair, he realized that he could have a great sexual relationship with someone along with other aspects of a romantic relationship. This left Evan no choice: he filed for divorce and began the process of finding a new partner who would better fit his needs, sexually and otherwise. He worked hard to minimize any damage to his preteen son and worked with his ex-wife to continue being the best parents they could.

Evan learned that denying his sexual side lead to years of blaming himself and not being realistic about the health of his marriage. Often people will convince themselves that sex is not that important or that they want it "too much" when their partner is a poor match for them because they want it too little. Evan had given into his wife's desires because he wasn't willing to stand up for his own. I often say, "If you are bending over backwards so far that you can kiss your own ass, you have gone too far." Evan is a good example of bending over too far.

A mix of emotions: What do these teach us?

Can you see the mix of emotions that weaves through each of our examples? Are you seeing any similarities to your own situation and life? David, Josh, Veronica, and Evan all experienced the Big Four emotions. Fear kept all of them from accepting their true sexual selves until circumstances forced them to face reality. Once they were forced to examine their needs and give themselves permission to explore, they understood how that fear was holding them back. They also realized how they had far more emotional strength than they imagined.

All of them experienced a lot of guilt as well. They felt guilty because they wanted and needed more from their sexual relationships, guilt for not sharing this side of themselves with those they loved sooner, and guilt for being less than perfect and making decisions that hurt those they cared about rather than facing these issues sooner in their lives. Part of being human is being an imperfect being. Learning to accept our own imperfection can be difficult for many people, especially those who want to do the "right thing."

Several of them felt shame and embarrassment. They felt embarrassed and ashamed that they were different from the people around them. Embarrassed that their sexual desires were deemed weird those few times in their lives when they were brave enough to disclose them. This shame and embarrassment made it easier to continue to hide this side of themselves until they could no longer do so. There was also deep shame for deciding to break the promise of an exclusive relationship.

Hopefully, these examples give you the information you need to keep you from making some of the mistakes they made. If you have already made some of these mistakes, hopefully these examples can serve as a way to handle those challenging and less than ideal situations.

Exercises: Field trips

Now is the time for exploration. Whether you're interested in BDSM, kinks, fetishes or an open relationship, now is the time to have some real-life experiences. It is impossible to know if this is the right path for you until you experience it for yourself. You cannot learn to drive a car by reading a book. You have to get behind the wheel and discover how it feels once the vehicle starts to move.

In many areas of the country, Meetup.com has groups of like-minded people such as polyamory groups. There are small local groups for kinks and fetishes and even national conventions that will allow you to see you are not alone. Many communities have local BDSM dungeons and swinger clubs. Even if you do not partake yet, meet other people who live these lifestyles, talk to them, ask questions, and learn as much as you can.

Once you have had a few experiences, journal about what you have experienced and your feelings associated with them. As we mentioned earlier, journaling can be a very powerful tool to help you examine any mixed feeling or emotions.

Check in: How are you doing?

Now that you have had some level of experience, what do you notice? Are you on cloud nine, excited beyond belief? Did that excitement then lead to the fear of some of the tough decisions ahead? Were your experiences positive, negative, or a mix of both? Are you more confused than before you started? Do you need further exploration to help you decide the best path?

You now have knowledge about how our society attempts to control your sexuality and education on alternative sexuality and relationship choices. Perhaps you've even had some real-world experiences. In Chapter 10, we will get to the tough choices. This may bring up much of your Big Four emotions again. Please remember, I am still here to guide and support you. Our journey is not over yet.

Chapter Ten

Now What?

Making the tough choices

"I can't believe s/he will ever accept this. How will I explain it? What if s/he leaves me? What if s/he wants a divorce? What am I going to do?" I have heard these fear-filled thoughts from multiple people in my practice and personal life as well as the people we discussed in the last chapter. All of them were terrified to talk to their spouses about their newly-accepted sexual wants, needs and desires, and none were sure how to explain what they wanted. While some discovered their spouse was eventually willing to renegotiate their sexual and relationship dynamics, others found they had to end their marriage and start over in order to be their true selves. This required the start of a journey to find a new partner who could accept and love all of them, including their unique sexual selves.

Learning to understand, accept and love your authentic sexual self may mean some tough choices and conversations with the people you care about. I will not lie to you; this is often the most difficult part and usually the part which people dread most. It is these very conversations and choices that have kept people from expressing their authentic sexual selves.

Once you are fully honest with your partner about your needs, they may surprise you beyond belief. It is amazing how some of the most traditionally-tailored people are willing to re-negotiate their relationship dynamics to keep their relationship going. Other times, a partner can be so entrenched in societal beliefs, concerned about what others think, or have a sexual personality type incompatible with what you need that the relationship is impossible to save.

We will also examine situations where a partner is so rigid, controlling or vindictive that even telling them the reason the relationship is ending is counterproductive. While these situations may be difficult to recognize or even admit, it is important to be realistic, especially in cases of divorce and child custody where this information could be used against you.

If you feel your fear rising up at the moment, don't despair. You are probably stronger than you realize. Remember the old saying: what doesn't kill you makes you stronger.

Talking with your partner

The work you have done so far—learning to manage your negative emotions, building your self-confidence, and educating yourself about your desired area of unique sexual expression—was part of the process leading up to this point. Without all this preliminary work, the odds of success when talking to your partner would certainly be less. While this type of preparation cannot guarantee a 100 percent success rate, it gives you a much stronger position from which to start.

Realize that you may stumble and stammer as you begin these conversations. That is OK. What is important is that you start. It will most likely be multiple discussions, so be prepared. Depending on your partner's personality, s/he may want a lot of information up front or in smaller chunks so s/he can think about it, process it, then learn more and talk further.

I always recommend talking in some sort of neutral place. It is usually an extremely bad idea to start this conversation when you are both in bed attempting to be sexual, naked in the bathroom, or in some other equally vulnerable situation. If possible, talk alone at home at the kitchen table, in the living room, or leave the house and take a walk together. If you are working with a therapist you trust, find out if they are willing to have a joint session with your spouse so you can talk with a supportive person to help both of you process the discussion.

Be sure to have information for your partner to read and begin to educate themselves, yet be careful not to overwhelm them. Remember, you are ahead of them on this journey; they have to catch up. Do not expect them to immediately jump on the bandwagon. Patiently answer their questions and discuss their fears and concerns.

If things start to escalate in the discussion, it is best to take a break, calm down, and resume later. If your partner needs time to process this new information, give it to them. Try to agree upon a later time (an hour, day, or week) to continue the conversation. This is rarely a quick process, so be patient.

To integrate your new lifestyle or start over? That is the question.

Often when people are strongly engaged in their fear and convinced that their partner will never accept their new sexuality, they wonder which is the better choice. Should they work through a challenging integration process with their partner, or just start over?

There are many issues to consider before beginning this conversation with your partner.

You probably know your partner better than almost anyone else. If you have spent years together, you know how they tend to react in situations when everything goes smoothly as well as times when nothing goes as planned. How did they respond? Were they able to roll with the punches and figure out how to handle it? Did they shut down emotionally? Were they too rigid to deal with change? Did they become angry, blame others for the problem, or become emotionally or physically abusive?

It is important to be honest with yourself about what you and others have experienced from your spouse. This can make all the difference in the world as to whether to have the difficult discussion with them or end the relationship and start over.

If your spouse tends to be rigid, controlling, manipulative or they always need to be right, switch easily from "I love you" to "I hate you," or have a difficult time with perceived abandonment (even if it's not real), *seriously* think about your next move. Do any of these traits sound familiar? They can be signs of several difficult personality disorders.

People who have disorders like Borderline Personality Disorder, Narcissistic Personality Disorder, Antisocial Personality Disorder or Histrionic Personality Disorder are unlikely to handle relationship changes well. If you need information to better understand these disorders, CounsellingResource.com (http://counsellingresource. com/therapy/self-help/understanding) and Elements Behavioral Health (https://www.elementsbehavioralhealth.com/addiction-re-sources/mental-health-resources/understanding-personality-disor-ders-symptoms-signs) can help.

If you think your spouse meets the criteria for one or more of these disorders, I don't recommend sharing information about your alternative sexual desires with them. Others in my profession may disagree with me, but in my experience, personality disorders rarely improve, even with intensive therapy.

While it may seem extreme, I believe it is better to go ahead and end the relationship for another reason and start over. This is my professional opinion and you can take it or leave it. I have seen people with personality disorders react badly and adopt a scorched-earth "I will destroy you" mentality once they have information they can use to hurt you. Granted, these are extreme situations, but I have seen them happen and they do not end well.

Working through the process of integration

Since most people are not going to have the extreme personality disorders we just discussed, working through the process of re-negotiating the relationship and integrating your newly accepted sexual self is more likely to happen.

To give yourself the best chance for success once you start the conversation, it's important to gauge your partner's reaction. This should determine the speed at which you proceed. If their reaction is far more positive than expected, begin by sharing what you have been learning. They need to follow the same process you did: understanding how societal beliefs control people, learning to manage emotions, improving self-confidence, educating themselves about this unique lifestyle, then dipping their toes in the pool. Be patient with them and remember that you are a team. After all, if this is successful, it will not be because they are just doing it for you. Your partner needs to understand how they'll benefit from expanding their own sexual horizons.

Since alternative sexuality is an under-researched area, there are few statistics on the percentage of healthy people who desire to engage in different types of behaviors. The advent of the internet has shown a growth in many areas of alternative sexuality. More and more master's degree students and doctoral candidates are undertaking research on these subjects. It is possible that while your partner may not enjoy the same kink as you, once you open the discussion regarding your joint sex life, they may uncover their own kink to explore.

If your partner is less than enthusiastic about making changes to your sexual life, this may make for a slower process. This can be difficult; if you feel ready to go forward, the process of getting your partner on board can feel like going backwards. Remember the saying "slow and steady wins the race." Even if the process is slow, if there is progress, do not give up.

Do notice, however, if your partner is reluctant to move forward or appears to only be doing it for you. Remind them that they do not have to go on this journey with you. They always have the option to bow out, and each of you can start over with new relationships. While ending the relationship may not be the preferred choice, it is important to remind a reluctant partner that they are not being forced to engage in activities they do not want, believe in, or desire. Even if it is difficult, sometimes divorce/ending a relationship ends up being the best choice.

Forging a new path alone and searching for a new partner

If you do end your relationship and start over, there are ways to find a new partner who is more likely to embrace your unique sexual self.

First, make sure you take the time necessary to emotionally heal from ending your relationship. Divorce or the end of a long-term relationship can be one of the most stressful events people encounter in their lives. Do not underestimate the effect on your physical and mental health. One of the biggest mistakes people make when ending a relationship is to jump into another one because they feel lonely, afraid, or empty. These are uncomfortable emotions, and many want to run away from them and into the arms of someone, anyone, new.

This is the problem. If you haven't learned to stand on your own, you are likely to make the same mistakes that got you into a relationship with someone with whom you couldn't be your authentic self. Do you really want to have done all the work up to this point, only to have to do it all over again? As painful and uncomfortable as it can be, take the time to heal before starting over.

So how do you know how long is long enough before you start again? While there is no magic formula, the standard rule of thumb is one month for each year the relationship lasted. If you were together for 10 years, you probably have about a year ahead of you to heal. Depending on your personality as well as the dynamics of your previous relationship, that will vary. I once had an intense 14-month relationship; after it ended, it took me over a year to mend my broken heart. The one-month-per-year theory is just a starting point, and you will need to play it by ear. In my professional opinion, most people need a minimum of six months with the average being a year. Some people will need longer than that.

Once you are ready to find a new partner there are many ways to go about this. If you are seeking some form of open relationship, there are Meetup.com groups in many areas for polyamory discussion groups. These are not actual dating groups, yet many people are able to meet others who may be a good match as well as learn more about the dynamics of polyamory.

There are many websites designed for dating and meeting others seeking an open relationship, whether it is swinging, poly, or designer relationships. Some mainstream dating sites offer open-relationship options. Sites like Openminded.com, Plentyoffish.com, OKcupid.com, and Tinder are known for attracting open-minded people.

If you would rather be on a more traditional dating site such as Match.com, make your profile upfront about what you are looking for in a relationship without being blunt. This will weed out those who want strict monogamy or are not open to BDSM, kinks or fetishes. It will also help you find those who feel the same as you, or are curious. You could find someone who has never had the courage to try other options but is open to them. What a great opportunity to share what you have learned!

If you are looking for a partner open to BDSM, kinks or a fetish, many sites cater to these populations. While it's not an official dating site, FetLife.com is a wonderful way to find others who share your interests. Many romantic matches have come from meeting on this site. You can also attend local munches, discussion groups, or other classes designed to teach specific skills that will help you meet friends and possible partners.

Keeping you strong during this tough time

Whether you choose to integrate your new sexual lifestyle into your existing relationship or start over, this will be a challenging time. It is important to be kind to yourself during the stress you will be experiencing.

Going through this process will most likely trigger your Big Four negative emotions. Be sure to revisit the exercises in Chapter Two to keep them manageable. Also, remember the exercises from Chapter Five can keep your self-confidence steady. A reinforced self-confidence will go a long way toward keeping you strong during this tough time.

Now is also the time to maintain healthy habits like limiting alcohol and recreational drugs, eating healthy foods, and getting enough exercise. If all you want to do is hide under the covers of your bed or plop on the couch and watch reruns of your favorite shows, don't. Get up and take a walk. Call a friend and meet for coffee or tea. Take up a new hobby or learn to meditate.

Exercises

Making new lifestyle changes is a major decision that takes time and practice. Over the years, I have often used an analogy I like to call "learning to walk." For parents who remember the process of a child learning to walk, think back on that time. If you do not have children, you have probably seen one go through this process.

Human beings learn by making mistakes. It is the process of failing, trying the same thing again, and learning to make adjustments that teaches us the skills we need to master anything new. When learning to walk, young children go through the same trial-and-error process. Once children are a few months old, they sit and watch older children and adults walk and move about and begin mimicking their movements. Part of their failure to crawl and walk right away is because their muscles are not yet strong enough to hold them up. As they become stronger, they continue to try; rocking back and forth leads to crawling. Crawling leads to pulling themselves up on a chair or wall and standing. And standing eventually leads to their first steps and then falling on their diapered butts.

It does not dawn on a toddler to give up. They might cry a little, especially if they hit their heads when they fell, but soon they are back at it again. At no time do they feel humiliated or embarrassed by falling down. They have not yet learned these thoughts and feelings.

And no matter how many times they fall, they don't stop trying. Small children are just determined to succeed. Their thought is, "If all these other people can walk, I can too."

I tell you this because you are now an adult who has learned to feel at least somewhat embarrassed or humiliated about their mistakes. Too many people feel badly about making mistakes because they've forgotten that making them is how we learn. What you are about to embrace is a new way of living. You are going to make mistakes. It is how you will learn. Accepting your innate humanity will make this process easier. Be kind to yourself.

When you find yourself making an inevitable mistake, take a moment and notice how you have metaphorically fallen on your butt. If it is a big fall, let yourself feel sad, disappointed or whatever else you feel in that moment. Then get back up, brush yourself off, and try again.

Check in: How are you doing?

Making tough choices is the most difficult part of the process of embracing your new sexual self. It can be very easy at this point to second-guess your decisions and allow others to use guilt, fear and shame against you. If you have ever hiked up a mountain or large hill, it can often feel impossible to make it all the way to the top. Many people stop and turn around.

Look back on some of your previous journal entries. Remember what led you on this journey and what makes it important to you. You are getting close to the summit of your mountain. Keep your negative emotions in check, and let's push on to the top!

Chapter Eleven

Acceptance

Living with the new you

For the first year after Veronica and Michael settled back into their marriage post-separation, she came to me several times wondering if it would last. She feared he was doing this in order to stay married to her, and would want to return to monogamy one day. She told me that once while driving home after spending the evening with another man with Michael's knowledge, she worried that he may have become upset and changed the locks while she was gone. He appeared to be enjoying their new journey, but how could she be sure?

She got her answer when they decided to vacation at a lifestyle resort in Mexico called Desire. One afternoon they were in a large, 50-person hot tub mingling with other people from the resort. She had always known Michael was the outgoing sort who struck up conversations with people easily.

She was talking with someone in the hot tub when she realized her husband was no longer by her side. She looked over to find him performing oral sex on a woman on the edge of the hot tub. One woman became two, then three, until he had done this with five different women. Shortly afterwards, they went to their room to change for evening dinner. At that moment, she realized she no longer needed to worry; Michael had fully embraced their new lifestyle and had no desire to go back. She described the rest of the trip as sheer desire...no pun intended.

Once you have made the decision to live your new sexual life and be authentic, there are a couple of final steps in the process. In this chapter, we will focus on the process of learning to fully accept your new sexual self. Even if your partner has decided to continue with you on this journey, there can still be stumbling blocks as you fully accept yourself. From time to time, both of you may have doubts about whether this is the right path. If your partner is not fully integrated, you may find they are experiencing some resentment because life is now different. This can lead to some fear for you that they will eventually leave you because the new journey is "too hard."

Learning to adapt your sexuality mindset will take time; you will often feel awkward and sometimes question if you made the right decision. This a typical part of the process of fully accepting your new sexuality.

Let's wrap up of the journeys of David, Josh, Veronica and Evan. We will see how they managed to navigate their journeys and find their own definition of success. We will also examine your ability to accept yourself and truly feel comfortable in your own skin.

David: A unique Leather Family

When some in the BDSM community choose to create their own unique type of relationships that involve some of the dynamics of power exchange, they call their group of partners a "Leather Family." The meaning of the term varies for different people, but usually refers to those who understand and accept their BDSM lifestyle so they do not need to hide who they are or how they behave.

Early on in our work, David dreamed about having a Leather Family of his own. In his local BDSM community, he met others who had attained this relationship dynamic and envisioned what this could look like in his life. When we discussed it in his therapy sessions, he often feared that his wife would not go *this far*, and would leave him if he pushed for more. They had already negotiated the option for him to have another sexual partner who shared his BDSM desires. It often felt like too much to ask for more.

While David had no problems expressing his true Dominant nature with his submissive partner, he often struggled to be authentic and strong when engaging with his wife. He often allowed his fears and guilt to overwhelm him, and he assumed she would not be willing to discuss further negotiation.

This is an example of a level of partial acceptance people often struggle to overcome. If one doesn't fully accept their new sexuality, they will self-sabotage themselves in little ways. To be fully successful, one needs to learn to overcome this and move on to full acceptance of their authentic sexual self.

Luckily, David was able to do this. In time, he decided he wanted to buy another house for his submissive to live in near he and his wife. His submissive would pay rent to cover the cost of the additional mortgage. When he approached his wife, she was willing to accept this additional change to their relationship. For several years, the three of them had gone to dinner together and shared holidays. His wife had realized that David's new partner did not replace her. She learned that in many ways, she continued to enjoy the marriage they had always had. It was just a little different.

In the future, David hopes to find a second sexual submissive to live in the new house with his first submissive. Finding the right person to complete his Leather Family is not an easy task. He is taking his time to find just the right personality to fit his vanilla wife and his other sexual submissive. He has now fully accepted his authentic sexual self, so I would not be surprised when someday he tells me he has found her.

Josh: A new love who enjoys his fetish

Once Josh's divorce was final, he took a break from therapy to heal from his divorce before he sought a new relationship. Like many who enjoy fetishes, Josh often verbalized his fear that he would never find a woman who would enjoy his foot and shoe fetish. We had talked at length about being upfront about his desires and how to educate a possible new partner about his fetish while managing his negative emotions and keeping his confidence strong.

I heard back from him after just under a year. Josh wanted to come in to talk about the new woman he was dating. He reported that he had met her at a happy hour with some co-workers. They hit it off right away, had many things in common, and their conversations easily flowed.

Josh used the strategies we had discussed and began to drop hints about his unique sexual interests. This was not on the first date, but not too far into the relationship either, so they had time to make a connection before having the discussion. Much to his happy surprise, she not only was open to his foot and shoe fetish, she had a few kinks of her own that she was willing to share with him! Josh was excited beyond belief that he had met a woman who not only accepted his fetish, but met his other relationship needs.

The reason he returned to therapy wasn't just to share his excitement. There were some complications, and he needed help to understand whether he should continue in their relationship or move on. She was still technically married, though separated, and was slow to make the final decision about whether to file for divorce from her husband. Josh loved this woman and she loved him, so it was difficult to think about leaving and starting over yet again. However, he knew he could not wait forever.

In time he ended this relationship since his partner would not make a decision about divorcing her husband. His acceptance of himself and his unique sexual desires gave him the strength to pursue a relationship that embodied what he desired sexually and provided the other aspects he needed from a romantic partner. Previously, he would have accepted what little he could get and been thankful for it. Now he was able to be strong and realize he deserved to be truly happy and not accept second best.

Veronica: Integrating her husband into a new open marriage

Veronica and her husband, Michael, were happy to be back together. While not perfect, their sex life had improved and they were enjoying the exploration of swinging together. Since Veronica had a head start, she initially was his guide. However, it was not long before he learned what he needed and both partners were on equal footing in their new sexual adventure. They made friends in their local swinger community by attending parties and events.

What some people do not understand is that the official swinger community is about more than just sex. It is a social community and many of the events offered opportunities to meet other like-minded people, see if there was mutual attraction, and if so, meet again at a later time. There were also people they met with whom they were never sexual, but they enjoyed having friends who understood and shared their lifestyle.

150 NO MORE HIDING

They learned they trusted each other completely, did not fear the other would leave them for someone else, and were strong enough in their self-confidence, that issues of jealousy and envy were easy for them to discuss and work through. This eventually led them to begin teaching swinger 101 classes to those new to the lifestyle as a way to give back to people joining the swinger community.

Many of their sexual interests were different from each other, and their levels of libido remained further apart than either would have preferred. Rather than judge or feel resentful that they were not able to bridge this gap, they allowed each other to be true to themselves and find outlets for needs the other couldn't meet. They also discovered that by giving one another the freedom to just be, rather than resent their differences, they gained a deeper level of emotional intimacy and connection than they'd had previously in their marriage.

Michael, who had always been monogamous and never considered other options, discovered that he was polysexual rather than the monosexual identity he'd accepted without question. This discovery came about one day when they were discussing what they would do if the other died. Since their marriage now felt very solid, they no longer thought about divorce, so the only way they considered being apart was through death. Not intending to be morbid, the discussion lead them to discover that if either had to find a new partner, they wanted to stay in some form of open relationship. Going back to monogamy was no longer an option for either of them.

Now, more than fifteen years since their separation and successfully living in the swinging lifestyle, their marriage is stronger than ever.

Evan: Finding a new like-minded partner after divorce

Evan found himself in a bit of a quandary after his divorce and the end of his relationship with Veronica. What he learned about himself and his needs, both sexual and otherwise, left him with great information, but no one with whom to share it.

Men who have experienced the swinging lifestyle with a partner have difficultly continuing to swing if their relationship ends. Some swinging communities are open to single men, but others are hostile. Evan's community was not unfriendly to a single man, but it wasn't completely welcoming either. He was fortunate to have been accepted into the community as part of a couple, so even though that relationship was over, he had an easier transition than someone coming in without that experience.

He knew he wanted someone who could embody both the stability of his former marriage and the sexual variety he had discovered during his affair with Veronica. At first this appeared to be a tall order, and he feared he might have to compromise or wait a long time to find what he was seeking.

Even went back to the basics and started attending swinger events that were more about meeting and getting to know people than just straight sex. He met several single women and eventually someone with whom he clicked on all the levels he needed. She also had been engaged in the swinger community and was seeking the same level of commitment and stability while enjoying the variety each wanted. They moved in together within a year; several years later, they got married.

Evan learned that like Josh, he needed to remain strong after his divorce and not jump into any relationship that might feel good for the short run. He knew he needed to find the best match on all levels and not return to accepting relationships that offered far too little, as he had done with his ex-wife.

Learning to accept you

I hope you see important patterns in our examples. The process of learning to fully accept your new sexual self does not happen overnight. Whether you integrate your partner or search to find a new one, this process demands all the information we discussed in the previous chapters. The people in our examples had to learn to manage their negative emotions; this was not a one-time event, because these emotions needed to be addressed and managed from time to time, depending on the challenges that arose.

They also needed to maintain their confidence to have continued open communication with their partners. This confidence also served them well as they gained knowledge of their new lifestyle and learned more about themselves and those around them. It allowed them to hold firm to their belief that this was the right path, even when they wondered if it would be worth it. Their confidence also gave them the patience to keep moving forward even when progress was slow and they were unsure if they would reach their desired goals.

These are the lessons I want you to learn from these examples. Understand that it will take time and you will sometimes question if you are on the right path. It is OK to question it and have doubts. You will know this is the right path when the thought of going back to your old way of living seems more difficult than going forward.

Exercises

In the acceptance stage, fear and anxiety can easily return, so you will need to work on managing them. Continuing to manage your negative emotions and keep your self-confidence strong will solidify your acceptance of your new sexual self.

Since journaling can be a powerful tool when making big lifestyle changes, we will have you journal like you have several times during this process. If it's helpful to look back at some of your earlier journaling, go ahead. If not, continue to write down your thoughts, feelings, fears, hopes, and dreams. It can be helpful to focus your journaling on areas where your negative emotions flare up. Are there any areas where you still feel stuck in being able to accept your authentic sexual self? Notice these areas and see where this leads you.

Check in: How are you doing?

At this point, you are moving from walking to running. While success is much more likely, you are still capable of stumbling and falling. If you fall, don't worry. Assess the situation, get back up and continue. If necessary, be more aware of the areas you have tripped over so you don't repeat the same mistakes. In our last chapter, we will talk about the final step in the process: owning your new sexual self and loving the new you!

Chapter Twelve

Loving the New You!
Loving yourself is the ultimate goal

As I look around the pool, I feel at ease and at home. Despite the scorching, 110-degree dry heat of Palm Springs in July, there is no other place I would rather be at this moment. I have been fortunate enough to come across a rare and unique group of incredibly fun, intelligent, open, and embracing people who are dear friends. We meet here once a year for our wild weekend.

And yes, by most of society's standards, what we do is pretty wild and different. We are a mixed group that includes people of various open-relationship styles, BDSM interests, kinks, fetishes and sexual orientations—pretty much everything we have talked about in this book. What we share is far more than the camaraderie or even the sexual acts we engage in. It is our shared sense that all of us have gone through a unique journey of self-discovery. While this journey has been sometimes painful, we have come out on the other side having attained the ultimate goal. We have gone beyond acceptance of our sexual selves; we truly own it and love ourselves. *This* is what I want for you.

I used to think that accepting one's authentic sexual self was the ultimate goal. In time, I have come to realize that acceptance is not enough. To fully integrate lifestyle changes, you must love yourself and truly own who you have become.

You do not need to be as open about your sexuality as some people choose to be. Not everyone in your life needs to know this side of you. But for the process to be complete, you must be able to stop hiding your authentic sexual self from your intimate partner(s) and most importantly, from yourself.

People who do not fully love themselves tend to attract people who keep them down, don't believe in them, and don't support them. Loving yourself is not the same as narcissism; that is a whole different animal. Someone suffering from narcissism has an overinflated sense of self-importance, an extreme need for others' admiration, and lack of empathy for other people. When you learn to truly love yourself, there is no need to apologize for who you are, what you like and desire, and consensual behaviors you choose to engage in. That is the difference.

In our final chapter, we will see how far you have come in this process, help you decide if you have more to learn, and find ways to continue to enjoy the journey while helping others who may be on this same path and can benefit from what you have already learned.

Look back and see how far you have come

After a journey like the one you have been on, it is helpful to look back and appreciate how far you have come. The process doesn't happen overnight, so some of the changes you have been through thus far are subtle and may not be obvious to you. Think back to where you were when you first picked up this book and began to read. Do you remember your level of fear? The guilt and shame you felt for even considering such changes? The embarrassment to admit, even to yourself, that this side of you existed?

How far you have come also depends on where you are at in the process. If you read this book straight through without engaging in the exercises or making any changes, it is still rather academic. If this is the case, it's okay. Work through this process at your own pace. Some people go through it rather quickly, for others, it can take years. Still others struggle to get through it at all.

Even if you never make it to truly owning and loving your sexual self or attain greater skill in managing your negative emotions, building your self-confidence and gaining knowledge in the areas of unique sexuality can be a success. No matter what level you have attained so far, be sure to give yourself credit for the work you have accomplished up to this point.

Notice the present and appreciate it

Let's assess where you are in your journey. If you have not gotten to the point of fully owning and loving your new sexual self, do not fret. As I hope you understand from what we have discussed thus far, this is a process.

As we learned earlier in the book, many cultural expectations and belief systems use shame and other methods to control people with unique sexual behaviors. I realize that I may come across as being very opposed to our society. That is not entirely true. I am very critical of those who want to control the consensual sexual behavior of other adults, because they do not share those desires or take the time to understand others who feel differently from them. I am not out to convert anyone who is truly content in their sexual world. To be honest, I am quite happy for them. The problem I have is with those who believe that everyone needs to be in the same sexual box, that there is only one right box, and anyone who falls outside of it needs to be fixed or cured.

I often tell people that I feel a need to apologize for my profession of psychotherapy. Unfortunately, there remain a number of people in this field who believe in pathologizing unique sexual behavior as wrong and in need of treatment. Thankfully, increasing numbers of therapists think more openly than the way most of us were trained.

Where are you now? Are you at the point of loving yourself, or are you still struggling with acceptance? Wherever you are in your process, I want you to notice your current position. Please do not emotionally beat yourself up if you are not as far along as you think you should be. Notice what has changed. Even if you are simply more aware of societal pressures that keep you from being your true self, that is a step. Be cognizant of where you are now. I want you to appreciate it.

Appreciating where you are in the present moment is an important skill to have as you move forward. Once we have created a goal, we often forget to stop in the present moment to appreciate how far we have come, where we are, and how it feels in the moment. This appreciation can give you the energy and courage to keep going.

You also may want to assess if where you are now is as far as you need to go. Maybe your original goal was more than you need. Your journey is unique to you, just like it is for everyone else. There is no right or wrong, and there are many shades of variation along the way. Part of noticing and appreciating where you are now is so you can decide if you even need to go further. Maybe you do and maybe you don't.

Try this brief exercise right now. I want you to close your eyes, take a few slow, deep breaths, allow your body to relax, and just sit for a moment. Think about how far you have come on the journey to evolve your sexual life. How does it feel in this moment? Is where you have gotten so far feel like enough? Is it further than you need to go, or are you feeling like you're only partway towards your goal and need more? Let yourself sit with this for a few minutes. See what you notice.

What more do you need to learn?

Reflect on that brief exercise. If you long for more, it is time to examine those thoughts and feelings. Think about the experiences you have had with your new sexual lifestyle. Is something missing? What do you need?

Some people may need to go back and do more work on managing their negative emotions. As we discovered in Chapter Two, these strong emotions have been part of you for many years. Learning to manage them can take time.

You will know if you need more practice with emotional management if you continue to have a lot of fights with your partner regarding this new path. Do you both continue to step on the landmines and then have a huge fight about it, rather than discuss things more or less calmly? That can be a sign you need more work on negative emotions as well as building your self-confidence like we discussed in Chapter Five.

For some people, a single book is not enough to learn these techniques; you may need the help of a skilled therapist or coach. Of course, you will need one who is knowledgeable about and accepting of unique sexual behaviors. Depending on where you live, this can be challenging. A couple of good resources are the National Coalition for Sexual Freedom (NCSF), which has a site for kink-aware

professionals   at   https://www.ncsfreedom.org/key-programs/
kink-aware-professionals-59776, and the American Association
of Sexuality Educators, Counselors and Therapists (AASECT) at
www.aasect.org. Not all AASECT therapists are kink-friendly, so
read the individual therapists' profiles carefully. Some people are
more comfortable with a sex or life coach than a psychotherapist.

Whether you choose a coach or a therapist, you need someone
specifically trained in sexuality. Unfortunately, the field of sex coaching is still new enough that there is not a website that lists coaches
who have been well-trained. Before hiring a sex coach, be sure to
interview them and review their education credentials in areas of
coaching, human sexuality, and sexology.

You may be doing well with your emotions and self-confidence.
Perhaps you just need more experience. Whether you desire BDSM,
kinks, fetishes or an open relationship, the experiences you have and
the people you meet in your unique community will affect where you
are in the process.

If you have had less than stellar experiences thus far, consider
searching for new people and groups. Think about what made your
previous experiences less than ideal. Was it the people you met? Was
it how you interacted with them? Was it a combination of the two?
Be honest with yourself about your own role and what might be
causing these experiences to go poorly.

Becoming skilled in BDSM or with some level of open relationships takes time, education, and practice. While practice may not
make you perfect, it can make you skilled. Be sure to put in the time
to learn and practice, practice, practice.

Look forward and plan for more

If after the brief exercise you did earlier, you realize you want
more, what does that look like? If you have gotten to the point of

loving your new sexual self, that could mean you are now in your zone and looking forward to more experiences within your new community of peeps. If you are still working on your level of self-acceptance, what do you need to help allow you to continue to grow?

Visualize the next goal in your journey. What steps are necessary to achieve this goal? People tend to keep their goals in their head rather than write them down in black and white. However, studies show that people who write down their goals have a substantially higher chance of success. Writing down your goals and the steps needed to attain them does not mean they are written in stone. They can evolve with you.

There are many opinions on the best way to write your goals. I have seen methods of accomplishing this with anywhere from four to twelve steps. Here is a simple plan that can be very effective:

1. Identify your goal—write it down
2. Set a deadline— decide on a date when you want it complete
3. List obstacles—what could get in your way?
4. Identify people who will help you achieve your goal
5. Skills—list the skills you need to reach your goal
6. Plan of action—develop the steps to get there
7. Benefits—how will you benefit from achieving this goal? ("Seven steps of goal setting")

The steps involved in achieving a goal—or the goal itself—often need to be adjusted as you move towards it. This is because as you learn and grow, you will change in the process of working toward your goal. You may realize the original goal was not quite what you imagined and it needs to change.

Pay it forward: Helping others

To help you finalize the process of loving your new sexual self, it can be very helpful to pay it forward and give back to others with what you have learned so far. You do not need to be an expert in order to share your knowledge. Whether you are in a large or small community, you can set up and lead a discussion group if none currently exists. Even if you think you're the only one who feels as you do in your community, it's likely you are not. You may even meet someone who has more experience in your particular sexual area who would be willing to join you as a co-leader. Both of you can learn from each other and teach others.

Just as Veronica and her husband taught swinger 101 classes, you could offer something similar. Whether it is swinging, poly, or designer relationships; a class, discussion, or a support group, teaching others to navigate a unique relationship style can be very helpful for new people wanting to explore. You will be amazed by not only how much you know, but how much you can learn by sharing your current level of knowledge and hearing how they handled their own experiences.

If you have learned BDSM techniques like the intricacies of rope bondage, spanking or flogging, or gotten into the mental mindset of power exchange, you can share these as excellent training for newer people. Few communities have support or discussion groups for kinks or fetishes. These groups can be extremely important not only to help increase people's knowledge, but also as a way of forming a safe place for people to discuss and explore their unique sexual interests. Creating this type of community can help lessen the isolation that often affects people with unique kinks and fetishes.

Integration

Accepting and learning to love your new sexual self comes down to the process of integration. While the theory is that it takes 21 days for a behavior to become a habit, scientific studies show something different. Depending on the difficulty of the behavior, it actually takes between 18 and 254 days for new behaviors to become a habit, with an average of 66 days. In reality, it can take anywhere from two to eight months. Even if you are not 100 percent consistent with the new behavior, it can still build the habit over time. (Clear, 2017)

In time, a new habit becomes part of your personality, which is how integration works. Whether it is exercising regularly or working towards the integration of your new sexual self, time and persistence can turn new behaviors into regular habits. Those habits integrate and become part of who you are. While it may feel difficult, do not give up; keep moving forward. Even if you are not doing it perfectly, you will achieve your goal with persistence.

Exercises

At this point you have done the exercises and journaled your thoughts, feelings, and goals. Now it is time to celebrate. You may want to create a ritual or celebration to mark this milestone. It is important to celebrate all the work you have done, the various ingrained beliefs you have tackled, the emotions you have learned to manage more effectively, and the improvements to your self-confidence. You have learned that this was not a journey for the meek, but one for those who are much stronger than they ever realized.

Create your own way of celebrating this journey. Maybe it is with a piece of art, a tattoo with personal significance, throwing a party with your new community of friends, or even high-fiving yourself in the mirror. Celebrate and congratulate yourself for what you have accomplished.

Check in: How are you doing?

Congratulations! You made it. As we have discussed throughout this book, there will be ups and downs as you continue on the path of becoming your new sexual self. After all, this is no different than any other area of life, and you will have times of both great joy and of challenge. Thank you for allowing me to be your guide, tutor, and mentor.

Postscript

Once again, I want to thank you for going on this challenging journey of sexual enlightenment. It is not the right voyage for everyone, but it can bring amazing levels of personal power to those it calls.

I mentioned earlier that a single book, while designed to give you the basics of what you need to complete this journey, may not be enough. If you need a coach or therapist to help you further on your journey, I have given you some resources to find competent professionals in your area.

I have discovered that after going this far together, some people do not want to continue this journey with someone new and want to continue working with me. If this is you, I would be flattered and honored to help you as you continue on your journey. While my office is located in the Denver metro area and too far for many to travel, modern video conferencing gives us other options. If you are interested in continuing to work with me, feel free to check out my website at www.drrhoda.com. You will find options for continuing our work together.

If you just want to drop me an email to let me know about your progress, I would love to hear from you.

Acknowledgments

Writing a book is a solitary act, publishing a book is not. In the words of Hillary Clinton, "it takes a village." There are many people involved in the successful process of taking this book from an idea in my head to the product you now hold in your hands, and I need to thank them for all their amazing help along the way.

First, to Polly Letofsky, of My Word Publishing, and her wonderful staff. Thank you for your guidance, your expertise, as well as your delightful sense of humor!

To my writing coach and editor, Bobby Haas, for taking my sometimes random thoughts and helping me put them in a form that made sense to others. I am forever grateful for your encouragement when I needed it most.

To Victoria for the beautiful cover art, Micah for your keen eyes with proof editing and Andrea for all the beautiful formatting. So many details, so effortlessly handled.

To my wonderful husband, Andy. Your support, love, and patience (especially during the rough weeks this past summer when I was in the midst of writing and wasn't always my "best self.") I always know I can count on you.

To the many men and women who have trusted me with the most intimate parts of their lives throughout my career. You have all taught me so very much in life and made this book possible.

Thank you to my parents for a lifetime of love and support and teaching me to care about the lives of others. You gave me a desire to do more than just exist; you taught me to give back to the rest of the world.

Finally, to my business strategist, Kimberly Alexander: thank you, thank you, thank you! This book would not be possible without your tutelage, guidance, support, and belief in me. It has been a wild ride, and I suspect there is much more to come.

References

Aaron, M. (2016). "The authentic self: Resolving internal shame." *Modern Sexuality: The Truth About Sex and Relationships* (p. 109). Lanham, Maryland: Rowman & Littlefield.

Britten, R. (2001). "What is fear?" *Fearless Living: Live Without Excuses and Love Without Regret* (pp. 20). New York: Berkley Publishing Group.

Bullough, V., & Bullough, B. (1977). "Homosexuality, sex labeling, and stigmatized behavior." *Sin, Sickness and Sanity: A History of Sexual Attitudes* (p. 198). New York: New American Library.

Clear, J. (2017). "How long does it actually take to form a new habit (backed by science)." Retrieved from http://jamesclear.com/new-habit

Connelly, J. (2012). "Clinical hypnosis with rapid trauma resolution." *Clinical Hypnosis with Rapid Trauma Resolution: Level 1* (p. 34). Tampa, FL: Institute for Survivors of Sexual Violence.

Diagnostic and Statistical Manual of Mental Disorders (5th ed.). (2013). Arlington, VA: American Psychiatric Association.

Donague, C. (2015). "Why we're scared of sex." *Sex Outside the Lines* (pp. 29-30). Dallas, TX: Benbella Books.

Jeffers, S. (2007). *Feel the Fear...And Do It Anyway* (2nd ed.). New York: Ballantine Books.

Kashdan, T., & Biswas-Diener, R. (2014). "What's so good about feeling bad?" *The Upside of Your Dark Side* (pp. 60-61). New York: Plume.

Klein, M. (2006). *America's War on Sex*. Westport, CT: Praeger Publishers.

Kort, J. (2006). "Straight men who have sex with other men." Retrieved from www.joekort.com

Lamia, M. (2011, December 20, 2011). Embarrassment [Blog post]. Retrieved from https://www.psychologytoday.com

Ley, D. J. (2012). *The Myth of Sex Addiction*. Lanham, MD: Rowman & Littlefield.

Maxmen, A. (2007, October 26, 2007). "Secret shame [magazine]." *Psychology Today*. Retrieved from http://www.psychologytoday.com/articles/200710/secret-shame

McDermott, E., Roen, K., & Scourfield, J. (2008, November 2008). "Avoiding shame: young LGBT people, homophobia and self-destructive behaviors [Article]." *Culture, Health & Sexuality, 10* (8), 815-829. http://dx.doi.org/10.1080/13691050802380974

Michaels, M. A., & Johnson, P. (2015). *Designer Relationships: A Guide to Happy Monogamy, Positive Polyamory, and Optimistic Open Relationships*. Jersey City, NJ: Cleis Press.

Onofrey, D. C. (2017). *Your Relationship with You: How to Live Life by Your Rules*. Greenwood Village, CO: AugustFirst Publishing.

Reivich, K., & Shatte, A. (2002). "Learning your ABC's." *The Resilience Factor* (p. 83). New York: Three Rivers Press.

Segal, J. (1997). "It's smart to feel." *Raising Your Emotional Intelligence* (p. 13). New York: Henry Holt and Company.

"Seven steps of goal setting." Retrieved from occonline.occ.cccd.edu/online/klee/GoalSetting.pdf

Schermer Sellers, T. (2017). *Sex, God & the Conservative Church*. New York: Routledge.

Shame, definition [Google comment]. (2017, May 10, 2017). Retrieved from http://www.google.com/?gws_rd=ssl#q=shame+definition

Taverner, W. J. (Ed.). (2008). "Sex addiction: Recovering from a shady concept." *Taking Sides: Clashing Views in Human Sexuality* (10th ed., pp. 11-17). Dubuque, IA: McGraw Hill.

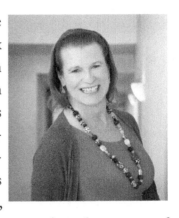

About the Author

Dr. Rhoda Lipscomb is an Alternative Sexuality Specialist, Certified Sex Therapist, and Clinical Sexologist with her PhD in clinical sexology. She is an author, teacher, public speaker and has been counseling and consulting with individuals and couples in the area of human sexuality for over 25 years. She has been the guest expert on several podcasts, teaches in a sex therapy certification program, and speaks on areas of alternative sexuality. She is an AASECT certified sex therapist with an ASCH certification in clinical hypnosis.

Dr. Lipscomb specializes in alternative sexuality communities such as open relationships, GLBTQ, BDSM, ABDL, kinks and fetishes. Her approach to therapy focuses on helping people understand, accept, and appreciate their sexuality with all its unique flavors.

To find more information or to hire her to speak at your event, contact her at her website: www.drrhoda.com.

Made in the USA
Middletown, DE
01 August 2020